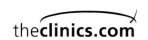
theclinics.com

PEDIATRIC CLINICS
OF NORTH AMERICA

Performance Enhancing Drugs

GUEST EDITORS
Peter D. Rogers, MD, MPH, FAAP
Brian H. Hardin, MD

August 2007 • Volume 54 • Number 4

SAUNDERS

An Imprint of Elsevier, Inc.
PHILADELPHIA   LONDON   TORONTO   MONTREAL   SYDNEY   TOKYO

W.B. SAUNDERS COMPANY
A Division of Elsevier Inc.

1600 John F. Kennedy Boulevard • Suite 1800 • Philadelphia, Pennsylvania 19103

http://www.theclinics.com

THE PEDIATRIC CLINICS OF NORTH AMERICA
August 2007
Editor: Carla Holloway

Volume 54, Number 4
ISSN 0031-3955
ISBN-13: 978-1-4160-5108-4
ISBN-10: 1-4160-5108-2

The ideas and opinions expressed in *The Pediatric Clinics of North America* do not necessarily reflect those of the Publisher. The Publisher does not assume any responsibility for any injury and/or damage to persons or property arising out of or related to any use of the material contained in this periodical. The reader is advised to check the appropriate medical literature and the product information currently provided by the manufacturer of each drug to be administered to verify the dosage, the method and duration of administration, or contraindications. It is the responsibility of the treating physician or other health care professional, relying on independent experience and knowledge of the patient, to determine drug dosages and the best treatment for the patient. Mention of any product in this issue should not be construed as endorsement by the contributors, editors, or the Publisher of the product or manufacturers' claims.

The Pediatric Clinics of North America (ISSN 0031-3955) is published bi-monthly by Elsevier Inc. 360 Park Avenue South, New York, NY 10010-1710. Months of publication are February, April, June, August, October, and December. Business and Editorial Offices: 1600 John F. Kennedy Blvd., Suite 1800, Philadelphia, PA 19103-2899. Customer Service Office: 6277 Sea Harbor Drive, Orlando, FL 32887-4800. Periodicals postage paid at New York, NY and additional mailing offices. Subscription prices are $138.00 per year (US individuals), $281.00 per year (US institutions), $187.00 per year (Canadian individuals), $367.00 per year (Canadian institutions), $209.00 per year (international individuals), $367.00 per year (international institutions), $72.00 per year (US students), $110.00 per year (Canadian students), and $110.00 per year (foreign students). To receive students/resident rare, orders must be accompanied by name of affiliated institution, date of term, and the signature of program/residency coordinator on institution letterhead. Orders will be billed at individual rate until proof of status is received. Foreign air speed delivery is included in all Clinics subscription prices. All prices are subject to change without notice. POSTMASTER: Send address changes to *The Pediatric Clinics of North America*, Elsevier Periodicals Customer Service, 6277 Sea Harbor Drive, Orlando, FL 32887-4800. **Customer Service: 1-800-654-2452 (US). From outside of the US, call 1-407-345-4000.** E-mail: hhspcs@harcourt.com.

The Pediatric Clinics of North America is also published in Spanish by McGraw-Hill Inter-americana Editores S.A., Mexico City, Mexico; in Portuguese by Riechmann and Affonso Editores, Rua Comandante Coelho 1085, CEP 21250, Rio de Janeiro, Brazil; and in Greek by Althayia SA, Athens, Greece.

The Pediatric Clinics of North America is covered in *Index Medicus, Excerpta Medica, Current Contents, Current Contents/Clinical Medicine, Science Citation Index, ASCA, ISI/BIOMED,* and *BIOSIS*.

Printed in the United States of America.

GOAL STATEMENT
The goal of the *Pediatric Clinics of North America* is to keep practicing physicians and residents up to date with current clinical practice in pediatrics by providing timely articles reviewing the state of the art in patient care.

ACCREDITATION
The *Pediatric Clinics of North America* is planned and implemented in accordance with the Essential Areas and Policies of the Accreditation Council for Continuing Medical Education (ACCME) through the joint sponsorship of the University Of Virginia School Of Medicine and Elsevier. The University Of Virginia School of Medicine is accredited by the ACCME to provide continuing medical education for physicians.

The University of Virginia School of Medicine designates this educational activity for a maximum of 15 *AMA PRA Category 1 Credits™*. Physicians should only claim credit commensurate with the extent of their participation in the activity.

The American Medical Association has determined that physicians not licensed in the US who participate in this CME activity are eligible for 15 *AMA PRA Category 1 Credits™*.

Credit can be earned by reading the text material, taking the CME examination online at http://www.theclinics.com/home/cme, and completing the evaluation. After taking the test, you will be required to review any and all incorrect answers. Following completion of the test and evaluation, your credit will be awarded and you may print your certificate.

FACULTY DISCLOSURE/CONFLICT OF INTEREST
The University of Virginia School of Medicine, as an ACCME accredited provider, endorses and strives to comply with the Accreditation Council for Continuing Medical Education (ACCME) Standards of Commercial Support, Commonwealth of Virginia statutes, University of Virginia policies and procedures, and associated federal and private regulations and guidelines on the need for disclosure and monitoring of proprietary and financial interests that may affect the scientific integrity and balance of content delivered in continuing medical education activities under our auspices.

The University of Virginia School of Medicine requires that all CME activities accredited through this institution be developed independently and be scientifically rigorous, balanced and objective in the presentation/discussion of its content, theories and practices.

All authors/editors participating in an accredited CME activity are expected to disclose to the readers relevant financial relationships with commercial entities occurring within the past 12 months (such as grants or research support, employee, consultant, stock holder, member of speakers bureau, etc.). The University of Virginia School of Medicine will employ appropriate mechanisms to resolve potential conflicts of interest to maintain the standards of fair and balanced education to the reader. Questions about specific strategies can be directed to the Office of Continuing Medical Education, University of Virginia School of Medicine, Charlottesville, Virginia.

The authors/editors listed below have identified no financial or professional relationships for themselves or their spouse/partner:
Kathleen Blake, MD; Robert T. Brown, MD; Sergio R. R. Buzzini, MD, MPH; Marcel J. Casavant, MD; Edward M. Castillo, PhD, MPH; R. Dawn Comstock, PhD; Joseph A. Congeni, MD; LaRae M. Copley, RPh, MD, PhD; Jennifer L. Dotson, MD; Robert W. Fitch, MD; Gary R. Gaffney, MD; Andrew J. M. Gregory, MD, FAAP, FACSM; Jill Griffith, PharmD; Brian Hardin, MD (Guest Editor); Caroline K. Hatton, PhD; Cynthia Holland-Hall, MD, MPH; Carla Holloway (Acquisitions Editor); Julie M. Kerr, MD; Andrew Kopperud, MD; Anthony Lattavo, DO; Robin Parisotto, BA; Thomas L. Pommering, DO; Peter D. Rogers, MD, MPH, FAAP (Guest Editor); Troy M. Smurawa, MD; and, Andrew Yates, MD.

The authors/editors listed below identified the following professional or financial affiliations for themselves or their spouse/partner:
Richard L. Hilderbrand, PhD has a 401k fund held by Quest Diagnostics.

Disclosure of Discussion of Non-FDA Approved Uses for Pharmaceutical and/or Medical Device:
The University of Virginia School of Medicine, as an ACCME provider, requires that all authors identify and disclose any "off label" uses for pharmaceutical and medical device products. The University of Virginia School of Medicine recommends that each physician fully review all the available data on new products or procedures prior to clinical use.

TO ENROLL
To enroll in the *Pediatric Clinics of North America* Continuing Medical Education program, call customer service at 1-800-654-2452 or visit us online at *www.theclinics.com/home/cme*. The CME program is available to subscribers for an additional fee of $195.00

GUEST EDITORS

PETER D. ROGERS, MD, MPH, FAAP, Section of Adolescent Health, Columbus Children's Hospital; and Clinical Associate Professor of Pediatrics, The Ohio State University College of Medicine, Columbus, Ohio

BRIAN H. HARDIN, MD, University of Arkansas Medical School, Department of Pediatrics, Arkansas Children's Hospital, Little Rock, Arkansas

CONTRIBUTORS

KATHLEEN BLAKE, MD, Clinical Instructor, Department of Pediatrics, The Ohio State University College of Medicine, Columbus, Ohio

ROBERT T. BROWN, MD, Professor of Pediatrics, The Ohio State University College of Medicine; and Chief, Section of Adolescent Health, Columbus Children's Hospital, Columbus, Ohio

SERGIO R.R. BUZZINI, MD, MPH, Chief of Adolescent Medicine and Attending Physician of Sports Medicine, Departments of Pediatrics and Orthopedics, Geisinger Medical Center, Danville, Pennsylvania

MARCEL J. CASAVANT, MD, Clinical Professor, Department of Pediatrics; Clinical Professor, Department of Emergency Medicine, The Ohio State University College of Medicine; and Medical Director, Central Ohio Poison Center at Children's Hospital, Columbus, Ohio

EDWARD M. CASTILLO, PhD, MPH, Research Associate, Department of Emergency Medicine, University of California, San Diego Medical Center, San Diego, California

R. DAWN COMSTOCK, PhD, Assistant Professor, College of Medicine, Department of Pediatrics; College of Public Health, Division of Epidemiology, The Ohio State University; and Primary Investigator, Columbus Children's Hospital, Center for Injury Research and Policy, Columbus, Ohio

JOSEPH A. CONGENI, MD, Associate Professor of Pediatrics, Northeastern Ohio Universities College of Medicine, Rootstown; and Division Director, Division of Sports Medicine, Akron Children's Hospital, Akron, Ohio

LaRAE M. COPLEY, RPh, MD, PhD, Clinical Instructor, Department of Pediatrics, The Ohio State University College of Medicine; and Resident, Department of Psychiatry, The Ohio State University Hospitals, Columbus, Ohio

JENNIFER L. DOTSON, MD, Pediatric Resident, Department of Pediatrics, Columbus Children's Hospital, Columbus, Ohio

ROBERT W. FITCH, MD, Assistant Professor, Orthopedics and Emergency Medicine, Vanderbilt University Medical Center; Team Physician, Vanderbilt University, Nashville, Tennessee

GARY R. GAFFNEY, MD, Associate Professor of Psychiatry, Division of Children and Adolescent Psychiatry, Department of Psychiatry, University of Iowa School of Medicine, Iowa City, Iowa

ANDREW J.M. GREGORY, MD, FAAP, FACSM, Assistant Professor, Orthopedics and Pediatrics; and Program Director, Pediatric Sports Medicine Fellowship, Vanderbilt University Medical Center; Team Physician, Vanderbilt University, Nashville, Tennessee

JILL GRIFFITH, PharmD, Certified Specialist of Poison Information, Central Ohio Poison Center at Children's Hospital; and Clinical Assistant Professor, The Ohio State University College of Pharmacy, Columbus, Ohio

CAROLINE K. HATTON, PhD, Consultant, UCLA Olympic Laboratory, University of California at Los Angeles, Los Angeles, California

RICHARD L. HILDERBRAND, PhD, United States Anti-Doping Agency, Colorado Springs, Colorado

CYNTHIA HOLLAND-HALL, MD, MPH, Associate Professor of Clinical Pediatrics, The Ohio State University College of Medicine; and Medical Director, Adolescent Medicine, Children's Hospital, Columbus, Ohio

JULIE M. KERR, MD, Clinical Assistant Professor of Pediatrics, Northeastern Ohio Universities College of Medicine, Rootstown; and Program Director, Primary Care Sports Medicine Fellowship Program, Division of Sports Medicine, Akron Children's Hospital, Sports Medicine Center, Akron, Ohio

ANDREW KOPPERUD, MD, Resident in Internal Medicine and Pediatrics, Columbus Children's Hospital; and The Ohio State University College of Medicine, Columbus, Ohio

ANTHONY LATTAVO, DO, Primary Care Sports Medicine Fellow, Grant Medical Center, Columbus, Ohio

ROBIN PARISOTTO, BA, Research Consultant, International Centre for East African Running Science, Glasgow University, Glasgow, Scotland

THOMAS L. POMMERING, DO, Clinical Assistant Professor, Departments of Pediatrics and Family Medicine, The Ohio State University School of Medicine; Medical Director, Sports Medicine Program, Columbus Children's Hospital; and Medical Director, Tour de Grandview Professional Cycling Race, Columbus, Ohio

PETER D. ROGERS, MD, MPH, FAAP, Section of Adolescent Health, Columbus Children's Hospital; and Clinical Associate Professor of Pediatrics, The Ohio State University College of Medicine, Columbus, Ohio

TROY M. SMURAWA, MD, Assistant Professor of Pediatrics, Northeastern Ohio Universities College of Medicine, Rootstown; and Division of Sports Medicine, Children's Hospital Medical Center of Akron, Akron, Ohio

ANDREW YATES, MD, Clinical Instructor, Department of Pediatrics, The Ohio State University College of Medicine; and Fellow, Division of Cardiology, Children's Hospital, Columbus, Ohio

CONTENTS

healthy behaviors. This article is intended to assist pediatricians by providing a summary of the current state of knowledge regarding the prevalence of use of performance-enhancing substances by United States adolescents.

Whether providing anticipatory guidance to the young adolescent patient, conducting a preparticipation examination on a young athlete, or treating a sick user of anabolic androgenic steroids (AASs), the primary care physician must be familiar with the adverse consequences of the use of these compounds. This article reviews the endocrine, cardiovascular, neuropsychiatric, musculoskeletal, hematologic, hepatic, and miscellaneous effects of AASs, highlighting effects reported in children and adolescents, and relying on consequences in adults when pediatric data is unavailable.

Dating back to the earliest Olympics, athletes have been searching for a performance edge. Recombinant human erythropoietin was made commercially available in 1987 to treat various diseases associated with anemia. Within a few years, elite endurance athletes capitalized on its potential as an undetectable performance-enhancing agent. Although antidoping agencies have developed a test to detect its use, there are pitfalls. More importantly, athletes continue to add more sophisticated doping practices to their armamentarium, challenging regulatory agencies, putting their health at great risk, and tainting the spirit of fair competition.

The presence of a prohibited substance in an athlete's urine (or blood, when applicable) or the use of a prohibited method constitutes a doping offense, even if the substance is a pharmaceutical and is properly prescribed. To avoid a doping offense for the therapeutic use of a prohibited substance or method the International Standard for Therapeutic Use Exemptions (TUE) must be followed. When the TUE is required, the appropriate process must be completed before testing under conditions where the substance or method is prohibited. This article describes the World Anti-Doping Code and the International Standards, which are part of the Code. In addition, the procedures for the proper preparation and submission of TUE requests are presented along with the manner in which the requests are considered by the Therapeutic Use Exemption Committees.

This primer on urine analysis in sports-doping control is an overview with an emphasis on the main analytical chemistry technologies in use: gas chromatography-mass spectrometry (GC-MS), liquid chromatography-tandem mass spectrometry (LC-MS-MS), isotope ratio mass spectrometry detection of exogenous testosterone use, and isoelectric focusing detection of recombinant erythropoietin (EPO) use. Included are graphic examples of GC-MS selected ion monitoring and full scan, LC-MS-MS, and EPO test electropherogram data; a list of common acronyms; and answers to questions frequently asked about tampering and test accuracy.

Ergogenic dietary supplement use is highly prevalent among adolescent and collegiate athletes, and use is increasing. To make appropriate recommendations for or against use by individual athletes, physicians who work with adolescent athletes should be knowledgeable about the most commonly used supplements and be able to access high-quality information about others. This article first discusses the legal and regulatory environment of dietary supplements. Several of the most commonly used supplements are then discussed in detail, including creatine, beta-hydroxy-beta-methylbutyrate, protein, amino acids, stimulants, alkalotic agents, glycerol, vitamins, and minerals. Finally, the "Gateway Theory" as it may relate to adolescent supplement and other drug use is discussed.

The history of anabolic-androgenic steroids (AASs) is an interesting tale that has its roots in ancient "endocrinology." More than 6000 years ago, farmers noted enhanced domestication of animals after castration. The development of AASs, and, later, their artificial synthesis, have remained a hot topic in scientific research and pharmaceuticals. Over the years, AASs have been used as a proposed treatment for a wide variety of ailments, despite deleterious side effects. Unfortunately, they have been, and still are, abused by body builders, athletes, and teens.

gaining a dishonest competitive advantage. Building on advances in genetics, a new threat arises from athletes using gene therapy techniques in the same manner that some abused performance-enhancing drugs were used. Gene doping, as this is known, may produce spectacular physiologic alterations to dramatically enhance athletic abilities or physical appearance. Furthermore, gene doping may present pernicious problems for the regulatory agencies and investigatory laboratories that are entrusted to keep sporting events fair and ethical. Performance-enhanced genetics will likewise present unique challenges to physicians in many spheres of their practice.

The underground abuse of growth hormone (GH) among young athletes presents a challenge to medical professionals. Health care professionals providing knowledgeable guidance regarding healthy ways to improve performance and appearance, as well as accurate information regarding substances' perceived benefits, risks, and unknown qualities, is invaluable to the young athlete. Further research focused on the profile and motivation of young people who use GH is essential to understanding and intervening better with those who use these substances.

FORTHCOMING ISSUES

RECENT ISSUES

ELSEVIER
SAUNDERS

PEDIATRIC CLINICS
OF NORTH AMERICA

Pediatr Clin N Am 54 (2007) xv–xvi

Preface

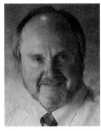 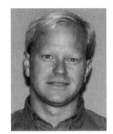

Peter D. Rogers, MD, MPH, FAAP   Brian H. Hardin, MD
Guest Editors

The use of performance enhancing drugs (PEDs) has become a burgeoning issue over the past few years. The use of these substances among both professional and Olympic athletes has filled the sports pages and incited the curiosity of our youth. Just how much these PEDs can improve athletic performance is not clear. And because there are so many PEDs on the open and black markets, those of us who take care of children, adolescents, and young adults have to be alert to the probability that our patients are exposed to these substances and may be using them.

Unfortunately there is a dearth of information in the pediatric and adolescent medicine literature on the use of PEDs in children and adolescents. Much of the information in this issue, therefore, is gleaned from the adult literature. The editors of this issue have tried to make the information as immediate and practical for those of us who deal with children and adolescents.

The articles in this issue of *Pediatric Clinics of North America* include (1) the prevalence of the use of PEDs among United States adolescents, (2) the office assessment of the adolescent who may be using these substances, (3) a history of the development of androgenic anabolic steroids, (4) consequences of the use of anabolic androgenic steroids, (5) the science of laboratory testing for PEDs, (6) the use of creatine by adolescents, (7) testosterone precursor use by adolescents, and (8) gene doping and the use of erythropoietin and growth hormone by adolescents.

What we have included in this isssue is the state of the art of performance-enhancing drugs as it pertains to adolescents. We admit that our knowledge of these drugs and the effects they have on adolescent stands only on the threshold. Some of the information at this time is speculative, but some of it is frightening and, clearly, dangerous.

Acknowledgment

Dr. Rogers would like to thank Lisa S. Blackwell, MLS, Serials/Research Librarian, Children's Hospital Library, Columbus, Ohio for her help in the preparation of this manuscript.

Peter D. Rogers, MD, MPH, FAAP
Adolescent Health
Children's Hospital
700 Children's Drive
Columbus, OH 43205, USA

E-mail address: rogersp@pediatrics.ohio-state.edu

Brian H. Hardin, MD
University of Arkansas Medical School
Department of Pediatrics
Arkansas Children's Hospital
800 Marshall Street, Slot 900
Little Rock, AR 72202, USA

E-mail address: hardinbrianh@uams.edu

ELSEVIER
SAUNDERS

Pediatr Clin N Am 54 (2007) 651–662

PEDIATRIC CLINICS

OF NORTH AMERICA

Performance-Enhancing Substances: Is Your Adolescent Patient Using?

Cynthia Holland-Hall, MD, MPH[a,b,*]

[a]The Ohio State University College of Medicine, Columbus, OH, USA
[b]Adolescent Medicine, Children's Hospital, 700 Children's Drive, Columbus, OH 43205, USA

Participation in athletic activities can benefit adolescents in numerous ways. In addition to keeping adolescents physically active, sports participation may enhance self-esteem, decrease stress, and encourage individuals to learn to work as a team; however, for some adolescents, the aim is not simply to enjoy sports participation but to win at all costs. They are not interested only in excelling as a team, but in striving to be the best as individuals as well. These adolescents may be at risk for using performance-enhancing substances to help them achieve their goals.

It is not only the high-level or "elite" athlete who may be attracted to these substances. For many, adolescence is a time of intense preoccupation with one's own body and body image. As puberty progresses, insecurities about a changing and growing body may lead an adolescent to consider using whatever means are available to attempt to alter his or her physical appearance. Coupled with the common perception among adolescents that they are unlikely to suffer negative consequences of their actions, this may lead adolescents to experiment with these substances.

The American Academy of Pediatrics defines a performance-enhancing substance as "any substance taken in nonpharmacologic doses specifically for the purposes of improving sports performance." This may include prescription medications, nutritional supplements, or illicit substances that individuals use to increase their strength, speed, or endurance or to control weight or alter body composition [1]. Several performance-enhancing substances are summarized in Table 1, along with selected positive and negative effects associated with their use. Virtually no research has been published on the effects or the risks of these substances in adolescents; therefore, this

---

* Adolescent Medicine, Children's Hospital, 700 Children's Drive, Columbus, OH 43205.
  E-mail address: hollandc@pediatrics.ohio-state.edu

pediatric.theclinics.com

Table 1
Potential effects of selected performance-enhancing substances

Substance	Potential benefits	Potential risks and side effects

Anabolic-androgenic steroids	Increased strength
	Increased lean body mass
	Less muscle breakdown
		Acne
		Hirsutism
		Gynecomastia
		Male pattern baldness
		Liver tumors
		Agitation/psychosis
		Virilization in girls
		Testicular atrophy
		Hypertension
		Premature closure of
		  epiphyseal growth plates
		Infertility
		Ligamentous injury
		Precocious puberty in
		  younger adolescents

Steroid hormone precursors (androstenedione, DHEA)	None proven	Increased estrogen levels
		  in boys
		Possible androgenic effects,
		  as above

Creatine	Increased strength
	Improved performance in
	  short, anaerobic efforts
	Weight gain
		Dehydration
		Muscle cramps
		Gastrointestinal symptoms
		Potential risk for renal
		  toxicity

Human growth hormone	No proven effects on performance Decreases subcutaneous fat	Coarsening facial features Hypertension Cardiovascular disease Impaired glucose tolerance
Diuretics	Weight loss Enhanced muscle definition	Acute symptomatic dehydration Electrolyte imbalances
Nutritional supplements	None proven	Unregulated substances Potential side effects vary

Abbreviation: DHEA, dehydroepiandrosterone.

information is derived from adult studies. More extensive descriptions of the individual substances may be found elsewhere in this issue.

A large national survey of adolescent children of nurses revealed that 4.7% of boys and 1.6% of girls reported the weekly use of some kind of product to build muscles or improve the body's shape [2]. Substances used included protein powders and amino acid supplements, creatine, growth hormone, steroids, and steroid precursors. Five to 8% of adolescents stated that they have used creatine [3,4]. In a survey of high school football players in several Wisconsin schools, 30% reported that they used creatine [5]. Ongoing studies that assess substance use and other risky behaviors in nationally representative samples of high school students suggest that approximately 3% of high school seniors have used anabolic-androgenic steroids [6,7]. Reported use is higher among boys than girls. Younger teens, including middle school and junior high school students, are nearly as likely as older adolescents to report having used steroids [8]. About 40% of high school seniors did not perceive a significant risk associated with the occasional use of anabolic steroids [7]; although it has not been studied, it is reasonable to hypothesize that younger teens are even less likely to understand the associated risks.

Therefore, those providing medical care for adolescents must be comfortable assessing adolescents for the use of performance-enhancing substances during sports physicals, at visits for sports-related injuries, and during routine health encounters. To be perceived as a credible source of information on this topic, providers must be knowledgeable about the specific substances in question and must acknowledge the potential benefits of using these substances in addition to the inherent risks. A "just say no" approach to counseling is unlikely to have the desired impact on an adolescent who is considering using these substances. By understanding the adolescent's goals and desired outcomes, it may be possible to help him or her achieve these outcomes by way of safer, more appropriate means.

Identifying the at-risk adolescent

Certainly, performance-enhancing substance use is most prevalent among athletes. The "typical" adolescent user of performance-enhancing substances is a male athlete who participates in a sport that demands high degrees of strength, power, size, or speed. He is more likely to use tobacco, alcohol, and other illicit substances as well [9,10]. The practice is more prevalent among football, baseball, wrestling, and gymnastics participants and those who engage in weight training and bodybuilding. Athletes who have reached a plateau in their training may turn to these substances to "break through" to a higher level of performance. Elite athletes, including those hoping for a college athletic scholarship or a career in professional sports, may use these substances to gain an "edge" over the competition. Young adolescents who already have specialized in a single sport year round, rather than engaging in a variety of athletic activities, may be on this pathway as well. Wrestlers and other athletes who need to meet certain weight requirements may use diuretics to achieve acute weight loss through dehydration; bodybuilders also may use such practices to achieve greater muscle definition before a competition.

Not every adolescent user of performance-enhancing substances fits this stereotype. More casual athletes, perhaps less informed about these substances, may believe that these substances are a quick fix or short cut to improved performance or muscle building. Those who are frustrated or unsatisfied with the results of the efforts they have made with their training may be tempted to try these products. Even nonathletes desiring an improved physique may try using exogenous substances as a means of changing their bodies. Those who are particularly body conscious, who look at "muscle magazines" and related media, and who express an interest in becoming more muscular are at increased risk [2]. Adolescents who are being bullied may feel the need to "bulk up" to defend themselves or to intimidate others and may turn to these substances to help achieve that goal. Use is not confined to older adolescents; it is well documented among adolescents in middle school as well [8].

Adolescents are likely to do that which they perceive as normative. Therefore, knowing teammates, competitors, or other athletes who use these substances or believing that use is widespread may increase an individual's likelihood of using [8]. There may be a general feeling of acceptability of the practice among fellow athletes, rather than any stigma associated with use. Many athletes may believe that they are well educated about the substances that they are using (perhaps better educated than their health care providers), that they understand the risks and benefits, and that they are making appropriately informed decisions about using them. Those who believe that there is little risk for getting caught or reprimanded for the use of performance-enhancing substances may have less hesitation about trying them.

Adolescents with any of the above risk factors should be asked about their use of performance-enhancing substances. Those who are under pressure from their parents, teammates, or coaches to succeed in their athletic endeavors or whose identity and self-worth are largely defined by their sports participation and performance may be at particularly high risk. Recent documented changes in weight or body composition also should prompt the clinician to inquire about use.

Interviewing the adolescent

Before discussing this or any other sensitive topic with an adolescent, the provider should clarify his or her confidentiality policies with the patient and parent. It is reasonable to assure the patient that information regarding the use of performance-enhancing substances will be kept confidential unless that use is putting the patient's life or health in immediate danger. Adolescents have a right to know what their providers intend to do with information obtained in confidence, and they are more likely to answer questions honestly if they believe that their privacy will be protected [11,12].

Depth of interviewing necessarily depends on the amount of time that the provider has to spend with a patient. In brief encounters, such as during a visit for an acute sports-related injury, a single, directed screening question, "Are you using any substances to improve your sports performance?" may be used. In longer encounters, a more prolonged conversation about sports participation may naturally lead into a discussion of performance-enhancing substance use. This may include an assessment of hours per week spent training and playing sports, specific training practices, and how important the adolescent feels it is to participate in and excel at his or her sport. The provider should inquire specifically about the adolescent's goals with regard to physique/body composition and sports performance, in the current season and in the long term (ie, are they anticipating a college or professional career in sports). Explore what, if anything, the adolescent sees as limitations or barriers to achieving these goals and what they have done or considered doing to try to overcome these obstacles.

A technique of "indirect questioning" may put an adolescent at ease when approaching sensitive topics. Using this technique, the provider begins by asking the adolescent his or her thoughts on a topic in general or as it applies to other people. Gradually, the questioning becomes more and more personal, ultimately culminating in a discussion of the adolescent's individual beliefs and experiences. For example, one may begin by asking adolescents how they feel about the practice of "doping" in professional sports and if they think that it is acceptable for younger, amateur athletes to use any or all of these substances as well. One may then ask if the adolescent is aware of any people their own age, perhaps even their own teammates, who engage in this practice. Finally, one can ask whether the adolescent has used any of these substances. This indirect technique gives the provider the opportunity to demonstrate an open, nonjudgmental consideration of this information, thereby making it more likely that the adolescent patient will feel comfortable disclosing his or her own beliefs and behaviors honestly.

When patients disclose that they have used substances to enhance their performance or physique, the provider must ask appropriate follow-up questions to clarify the extent of use and assess the degree of risk associated with these behaviors. This line of questioning should include what doses of substances the adolescent is using and how this dosing regimen was chosen. If a nutritional supplement is labeled for use at a specific dose, an adolescent may take a "more is better" approach and use even higher doses. Adolescents' use of the jargon common to the world of doping may be a clue that they are at particularly high risk for engaging in more dangerous patterns of use. These patients may report "cycling" (using a substance for a specific period of time and then discontinuing use for a time, perhaps when anticipating drug testing), "pyramiding" (using a regimen of increasing and decreasing dosing), or "stacking" (using multiple performance-enhancing substances simultaneously). Patients should be asked where they get information about these substances (eg, teammates, coaches, Internet, nutrition supplement shops). The provider should ask about the presence of side effects and if the adolescent uses any additional substances to minimize side effects or mask detection of the substances they use, should they be tested for drugs. Patients who admit to using injection drugs should be asked about needle-sharing practices. Because adolescents who use anabolic-androgenic steroids are more likely to engage in other risky behaviors, they should be asked about the use of tobacco, alcohol, and other illicit substances as well [13,14]. Specific questions that may be used when interviewing an adolescent about performance-enhancing substance use, including indirect questions and follow-up questions, are listed in Box 1.

The physical examination

Most adolescents who use performance-enhancing substances have no distinguishing physical findings suggesting their use; however, a thorough physical examination may be useful in several regards. Height, weight, and body mass index should be obtained and compared with previous measurements. Body composition and degree of muscularity should be noted. Elevated blood pressure may suggest stimulant, human growth hormone, or anabolic-androgenic steroid use. In boys, anabolic-androgenic steroid use may lead to acne, male pattern baldness, gynecomastia, testicular atrophy, and severe striae. In addition to several of the above findings, girls may develop hirsutism, clitoral hypertrophy, and deepening of the voice. Injection drug users may have needle marks or evidence of skin abscesses. Creatine and other nutritional supplements are unlikely to have visible manifestations on physical examination.

Additional testing

Drug testing for exogenous substances may be performed, most commonly using gas chromatography with mass spectrometry; however, this testing may be of limited value. Availability of testing is limited, and some substances may not be detectable in a urine test. If urine testing is performed, the specimen ideally should be obtained under the direct observation of a same-gender member of the medical staff. If this is impossible, other measures to prevent dilution or contamination of the specimen should be considered, such as coloring the toilet water and disabling the sink in the restroom where the specimen is obtained. Although the threat or practice of routine drug screening may deter the "casual" user, a highly motivated athlete is likely to be one step ahead of the primary care provider with regard to techniques for hiding or masking his or her use. Furthermore, although such testing may limit the undesirable behavior, it is unlikely to lead the adolescent to give careful consideration to the issues of winning at all costs versus doing what he or she believes is morally right and justified. An open and honest discussion of the risks, benefits, and moral implications of doping may be more effective in this regard. A more extensive discussion of drug testing is contained elsewhere in this issue.

Patients who use injection drugs, particularly if they admit to any needle sharing, should be tested for hepatitis B, hepatitis C, and HIV. An electrocardiogram and metabolic profile, including glucose, a cholesterol and lipid panel, and liver function testing, may be considered in persons using human growth hormone and anabolic-androgenic steroids and their precursors. Electrolytes may be obtained in athletes who use diuretics or

Box 1. Questioning the adolescent patient about the use of performance-enhancing substances

Brief screening questions
- Are you using any substances to improve your sports performance?
- Are you using any substances to improve your body's appearance or strength?

Questions about sports participation and performance
- Are you satisfied with how well you do at your sport?
- What, if anything, do you think keeps you from being even better at your sport?
- Do you put a lot of pressure on yourself to improve your sports performance?
- Do other people in your life, like your parents, coaches, or teammates, put pressure on you to improve your performance?
- What are your short-term and long-term goals for sports participation (eg, plans to obtain an athletic scholarship)?

Questions about body image and satisfaction
- Are you happy with your current weight and body composition?
- Have you had any recent changes in your weight or body composition? How did you achieve this?
- Do you read magazines or visit Internet sites focused on bodybuilding or fitness?

Questions about performance enhancing substances
- How do you feel about professional athletes who engage in doping?
- Do you think it's okay for people your age to use substances to improve their sports performance? What kind of substances do you think it's okay to use?
- Do you think it's okay for schools to perform drug testing on their student athletes?
- Do you know any athletes at your school or on your team who use these substances? Which ones do they use?
- Has anyone ever encouraged you to use these substances?
- Have you ever used anything to improve your strength, physique, or performance?

Follow-up questions for positive screens
- Which substances have you tried? Which are you using currently?

- What dose do you use? Is this the recommended dose for this substance?
- Where do you get your information about using these substances?
- How did you determine the dosing regimen you use?
- Where do you get these substances?
- What changes have you seen in your body or performance since you started using this?
- Are you experiencing any side effects?
- Do you use any additional substances to help lessen these side effects or to avoid having a positive drug screen?
- Where do you get your needles? Do you share needles (if applicable)?
- Do you understand that it is illegal to use certain substances without a doctor's prescription?
- Do you use tobacco, alcohol, or any other drugs?

excessive quantities of creatine. Keep in mind that these laboratory values are normal in most athletes who use performance-enhancing substances; normal values should not provide reassurance that the adolescent is not using.

Prevention

Perhaps the most important role of the primary care provider is to discuss performance-enhancing substance use with adolescents before they consider or initiate use. Athletes should be encouraged to consider how they feel about competition, the importance of winning, and the importance of achieving their personal best performance. What constitutes fair versus unfair competition? How do performance-enhancing substances fit into this model of fair competition? Does the adolescent make a distinction between "legal" and banned substances in this regard? Patients who voice opposition to the use of these substances should be supported and their decisions reinforced. Skills to resist peer pressure to consider using should be taught, perhaps by way of role playing.

A categorical "just say no" approach to counseling is unlikely to be effective and may be detrimental. Recent media attention to doping in professional sports has contributed to widespread acceptance that the use of some substances does confer an advantage to the user. Some patients already may have seen beneficial effects in themselves or peers who are users. To be seen by the athlete as a credible source of health information, a provider must acknowledge that some substances, particularly anabolic-androgenic steroids, clearly have been shown to increase muscle mass and potentially improve performance. Creatine also has been associated with improved performance in some studies. The provider may proceed, however, by providing additional information about which some adolescents may not be aware. These two substances are only effective when used in conjunction with intense resistance training; they do not provide an effortless "short cut" to bigger muscles. Furthermore, they offer only a small benefit over a healthy diet and a rigorous training regimen. For the elite athlete, this may be the tiny edge that one needs over the competition, but the typical middle school or high school athlete may not perceive a significant difference in one's performance. The provider may point out that simple measures, such as getting enough sleep, maintaining adequate hydration, and quitting smoking, may have a greater positive impact on sports performance than using supplements. When discussing creatine use, adolescents need to be aware that approximately 20% to 30% of the population seem to be "nonresponders" who will not see beneficial effects [15]. Furthermore, the American College of Sports Medicine, while acknowledging the positive effects of creatine, does not recommend its use in persons younger than 18 years of age [16]. It is speculated, but not proven, that creatine may serve as a "gateway" drug, the use of which may lead to the use of more dangerous performance-enhancing substances.

Adolescents considering the use of anabolic-androgenic steroids need to know the potential medical risks and side effects associated with the use of these substances, including acne, striae, psychiatric symptoms, the development of liver tumors, and adverse cardiovascular effects. Female users may develop hirsutism, deepening of the voice, male pattern baldness, clitoral enlargement, and menstrual irregularities. They need to understand that some of the virilizing features may be irreversible. Boys may experience gynecomastia, hair loss, and testicular atrophy. Although the cosmetic effects may not be the most concerning risks from the provider's perspective, these concrete images, such as irreversible gynecomastia for a boy or hirsutism for a girl, may have a greater psychologic impact than more dangerous but more abstract risks, such as liver disease. Adolescents who are considering using steroids or other injection drugs should be educated regarding the infectious risks associated with sharing needles.

Many advertisements for performing-enhancing nutritional supplements are aimed specifically at the adolescent and young adult demographic. Some adolescents are becoming more media savvy and may respond well to the idea that those running the multimillion dollar industry of nutritional supplements are counting on young people to be vulnerable to their marketing claims. Remind them that these substances are not regulated by the US Food and Drug Administration in the same manner as prescription medications and that the claims made by advertisers often are not substantiated. Furthermore, quality control during the processing and packaging of these products is variable, and there is no guarantee that the contents of the container are reflected accurately on the label. Some products that are mar-keted as legal nutritional supplements conceivably may contain substances that are banned or dangerous to enhance their perceived efficacy. This could result in a positive drug screen or other adverse medical effects in an athlete who believes that he or she is using a safe substance. Of course, this also makes it impossible for the provider to counsel on the safety of these prod-ucts with any degree of certainty.

Counseling a patient not to take a particular course of action (eg, not to use performance-enhancing substances) is likely to be more effective if the provider can offer the patient alternative means of achieving the desired out-comes. Therefore, a broader discussion of an adolescent's motivation for considering the use of these substances is warranted. Ask the adolescent to describe his or her performance goals or goals for physical appearance. Help the adolescent to explore alternative ways to achieve these goals. Point out some of the adolescent's modifiable lifestyle choices that may be impair-ing performance, such as smoking cigarettes or marijuana, using alcohol, poor sleep habits, or poor conditioning. Become knowledgeable about local referral resources that may assist patients in making appropriate changes. Most adolescents have room for improvement in their diets; a sports nutri-tionist can help them to make better food choices to optimize their health and performance. The American College of Sports Medicine endorses the safety of strength training, even in preteenagers [17]; a qualified trainer can help them develop a safe and effective training regimen. Sensible weight control programs, such as Weight Watchers, are widely available in many communities and are appropriate for adolescents who wish to lose weight in a healthful manner. For adolescents with symptoms of a mood or anxiety disorder or who are experiencing stressful psychosocial situations, getting help from a mental health provider may enhance their overall well-being, which may be reflected by better performance in sports and other extracur-ricular activities.

Lastly, parents of adolescent athletes should be educated as well. Some may not appreciate the potential dangers of using certain performance-en-hancing substances; others may know that they can be harmful but may not realize how widespread their use is, even at the middle school level. Par-ents should know that the American Academy of Pediatrics strongly con-demns the use of performance-enhancing substances [1]. They should be encouraged to have ongoing discussions with their children, particularly those who are athletes, about this issue. These discussions become even more important as athletes aspire to higher and higher levels of performance in their sport. Parents should make their own views on the subject clear and communicate their expectations explicitly and repeatedly to their children. They should remind their children of all of the positive aspects of sports par-ticipation and encourage them to focus on these aspects and not solely on winning. They should attempt not to let their child's self-esteem be tied too closely to winning or performance and should encourage them instead to take pride in being fair and honest in their approach to sports participation. Parents should be aware of the side effects of dangerous substances and what to look for in their own child.

Summary

Adolescents have variable knowledge about performance-enhancing substances, but many athletes and nonathletes may be considering their use. Young adolescents are as likely as older adolescents to use these substances. Although most nutritional supplements are not likely to cause serious harm, they are largely unregulated and their safety cannot be assured. Anabolic-androgenic steroids, although illegal, are readily available to athletes who seek them out. Although the potential adverse effects of steroid use are unequivocal and should be emphasized, their positive effects must be acknowledged as well if a provider is to have a meaningful discussion with an athlete regarding their use. While discouraging the use of performance-enhancing substances, providers should be prepared to assist their patients in achieving their performance and appearance goals in alternative, healthful ways.

References

[1] Committee on Sports Medicine and Fitness. American Academy of Pediatrics. Use of performance-enhancing substances. Pediatrics 2005;115(4):1103–6.

[2] Field AE, Austin SB, Camargo CA, et al. Exposure to the mass media, body shape concerns, and use of supplements to improve weight and shape among male and female adolescents. Pediatrics 2005;116(2):e214–20.

[3] Metzl JD, Small E, Levine SR, et al. Creatine use among young athletes. Pediatrics 2001; 108(2):421–5.

[4] Smith J, Dahm DL. Creatine use among a select population of high school athletes. Mayo Clin Proc 2000;75(12):1257–63.

[5] McGuine TA, Sullivan JC, Bernhardt Dt, et al. Creatine supplementation in high school football players. Clin J Sport Med 2001;11(4):247–53.

[6] Centers for Disease Control and Prevention. Youth risk behavior surveillance – United States, 2005. Surveillance Summaries, June 9, 2006. MMWR Morb Mortal Wkly Rep 2006;55(No. SS # 5):16.

[7] Johnston LD, O'Malley PM, Bachman JG, et al. Monitoring the future national results on adolescent drug use: overview of key findings, 2005. (NIH Publication No. 06–5882). Bethesda (MD): National Institute on Drug Abuse; 2006.

[8] Faigenbaum AD, Zaichowsky LD, Gardner DE, et al. Anabolic steroid use by male and female middle school students. Pediatrics 1998;101(5):E6.

[9] Bahrke MS, Yesalis CE, Kopstein AN, et al. Risk factors associated with anabolic-androgenic steroid use among adolescents. Sports Med 2000;29(6):397–405.

[10] Kindlundh AM, Isacson DG, Berglund L, et al. Factors associated with adolescent use of doping agents: anabolic-androgenic steroids. Addiction 1999;94(4):543–53.

[11] Cheng TL, Savageau JA, Sattler AL, et al. Confidentiality in health care. A survey of knowledge, perceptions, and attitudes among high school students. JAMA 1993;269(11):1404–7.

[12] Ford CA, Millstein SG, Halpern-Felsher BL, et al. Influence of physician confidentiality assurances on adolescents' willingness to disclose information and seek future health care. A randomized controlled trial. JAMA 1997;278(12):1029–34.

[13] DuRant RH, Escobedo LG, Heath GW. Anabolic steroid use, strength training, and multiple drug use among adolescents in the United States. Pediatrics 1995;96(1 Pt 1):23–8.

[14] Middleman AB, Faulkner AH, Woods ER, et al. High-risk behaviors among high school students in Massachusetts who use anabolic steroids. Pediatrics 1995;96(2 Pt 1):268–72.

[15] Juhn MS, Tarnopolsky M. Oral creatine supplementation and athletic performance: a critical review. Clin J Sport Med 1998;8(4):286–97.

[16] Terjung RL, Clarkson P, Eichner ER, et al. The American College of Sports Medicine Roundtable on the physiological and health effects of oral creatine supplementation. Med Sci Sports Exerc 2000;32(3):706–17.

[17] Luebbers PE. The right time for kids to exercise. American College of Sports Medicine, ACSM Fit Society Page; 2003. Available at: www.ascm.org. Accessed May 30, 2007.

ELSEVIER
SAUNDERS

PEDIATRIC CLINICS
OF NORTH AMERICA

Pediatr Clin N Am 54 (2007) 663–675

Prevalence of Use of Performance-Enhancing Substances Among United States Adolescents

Edward M. Castillo, PhD, MPH[a],
R. Dawn Comstock, PhD[b,c],*

[a]Department of Emergency Medicine, University of California, San Diego Medical Center,
200 West Arbor Drive, #8676, San Diego, CA 92103, USA
[b]College of Medicine, Department of Pediatrics and College of Public Health, Division
of Epidemiology, The Ohio State University, Columbus, OH 43210, USA
[c]Columbus Children's Hospital, Center for Injury Research and Policy, 700 Children's Drive,
Columbus, OH 43205, USA

Undoubtedly, athletes always have striven, and will continue to strive, to improve their performance through means such as physical training, improved nutrition, and skills training. For thousands of years, the use of exogenous substances has accompanied efforts to improve performance by at least some competitive athletes [1]. In the past decade, the use of performance-enhancing substances by Olympic athletes and United States professional athletes has sparked a highly publicized discussion of the potential negative health effects and ethical implications of the use of such substances. The use of performance-enhancing substances has spread beyond the sporting arena, with increased popularity among individuals—nonathletes as well as athletes—seeking to improve their physical appearance. Annual sales of nutritional supplements (a broad term inclusive of some performance-enhancing substances) have been estimated at up to $12 billion in the United States [2].

Adolescents, who in the normal course of development become intensely concerned about peer acceptance, body image, and athletic prowess, may regard the use of performance-enhancing substances as an easy means to gain self-esteem through improved body appearance and athletic performance [3]. Additionally, normally experienced feelings of invulnerability can lead

* Corresponding author. Columbus Children's Hospital, Center for Injury Research and Policy, 700 Children's Drive, Columbus, OH 43205.
E-mail address: comstocd@pediatrics.ohio-state.edu (R.D. Comstock).

0031-3955/07/$ - see front matter © 2007 Elsevier Inc. All rights reserved.
doi:10.1016/j.pcl.2007.04.002   *pediatric.theclinics.com*

adolescents to use performance-enhancing substances with disregard to potential negative health effects and long-term consequences [3]. These are not new phenomena; the use of anabolic steroids by United States adolescent athletes reportedly occurred first in 1959 [4].

The use of performance-enhancing substances by adolescents is particularly troubling because safety data associated with the use of such substances by this population is largely lacking [5]. Most reports on performance-enhancing substances have focused on efficacy [6–9]. Few studies have focused on the use of these substances among adolescents; studies that have tended to focus on a single supplement. Additionally, published studies are difficult to compare because of the focus on varying ages, athletic backgrounds, selection variations, and analysis stratification. This poses a dilemma for the pediatrician who needs correct information, including the potential efficacy and negative health effects of such substances as well as the prevalence of use among adolescents and risk factors for use, to identify patients in need of counseling and to find the best way to help adolescent patients make informed decisions to promote healthy behaviors. This article is intended to assist pediatricians by providing a summary of the current state of knowledge regarding the prevalence of use of performance-enhancing substances by United States adolescents.

Overview of performance-enhancing substances

The term "performance-enhancing substance" is used commonly to refer to a broad array of agents that can be segregated into three main categories: illegal substances/substances not available without a prescription that are banned by some or all sports (eg, anabolic steroids and the hormone precursor androstenedione); legally available substances that are banned by some or all sports, in general or in competition only (eg, diuretics and caffeine); and legally available substances that are not banned (eg, dietary supplements). Determining the category into which a substance falls can be difficult because the lists of substances that are banned by the various sporting governing bodies are amended frequently. Also, although less frequent, a substance's legal status can change (eg, the US Food and Drug Administration's banning of the sale of supplements containing ephedrine alkaloids in 2004).

As detailed in the Dietary Supplement Health and Education Act of 1994 [10], "The term 'dietary supplement' means a product (other than tobacco) intended to supplement the diet that bears or contains one or more of the following dietary ingredients: a vitamin; a mineral; an herb or other botanical; an amino acid; a dietary substance for use by man to supplement the diet by increasing the total dietary intake; a concentrate metabolite, constituent, extract, or combination of any ingredient described above; is intended for ingestion in the form of a capsule, powder, softgel, or gelcap; or is labeled as a dietary supplement." The United States federal government allows for the manufacturing and marketing of these supplements with minimal requirements or regulation, and they are readily available at local markets and health food stores and from online retailers. Dietary supplements are consumed for a variety of reasons, including general health maintenance, increased muscle mass, and athletic performance enhancement. As with most behaviors, several factors contribute to the use of dietary supplements, including age and various health behaviors, such as smoking, alcohol use, and physical activity. In adolescents and adults, dietary supplements are becoming increasingly popular among individuals who are attempting to enhance athletic performance, improve body appearance, and achieve healthier lifestyles. This increase continues, despite the limited information on efficacy and safety for most products.

According to the US Anti-Doping Agency, a performance-enhancing substance gets placed on the prohibited list (ie, is banned by some or all sports) if it meets two of three criteria: it has the potential to enhance or enhances sport performance, it represents an actual or potential health risk to the athlete, or it violates the spirit of sport [11]. To aid athletes, the US Anti-Doping Agency annually publishes a *Guide to Prohibited Substances* that provides a list of substances banned in competition and out-of-competition by different sports' governing bodies. The US Food and Drug Administration determines the legal status of substances. Although these two categories of performance-enhancing substances traditionally have been used by athletes to improve performance, a growing number of individuals have adopted the use of such substances to improve body appearance.

In an effort to best serve the needs of the pediatrician, the review presented here has been limited to peer-reviewed publications that focused on performance-enhancing substances included in the US Anti-Doping Agency's *Guide to Prohibited Substances* [11] and performance-enhancing substances that are commonly available for purchase (eg, creatine), and large, unpublished surveys that assessed the prevalence of use of such substances by adolescents. In an effort to ensure the generalizability of results, the presentation of information not published in the peer-review literature is limited to national surveys. Thus, several state-based surveys capturing information on the prevalence of performance-enhancing substance use among adolescents were excluded [12–17].

Prevalence of use of performance-enhancing substances

Performance-enhancing supplement use in adolescents has not been studied adequately. Although there is a growing number of reports in the peer-review scientific literature on the prevalence of anabolic steroid and creatine use among adolescents, few reports provide information on the prevalence of use of other supplements. To provide an overview of the prevalence and patterns of performance-enhancing supplements in United States adolescents, pertinent peer-review publications focusing on these substances, rather than general supplement use, are summarized here (Tables 1 and 2).

Table 1
Anabolic steroid use among United States adolescents: reports in the peer-review literature

Investigators	Sample population	Overall prevalence
Buckley et al [18]	3403 male 12th graders	6.6%
Krowchuk et al [19]	295 high school athletes	1.0%
Johnson et al [21]	853 11th graders	11.1%
Whitehead et al [20]	3,900 10th–12th graders	5.3%
Radakovich et al [29]	810 7th graders	3.8%
Tanner et al [22]	6930 high school students	2.7%
Scott et al [23]	4722 middle/high school students	2.5%
Faigenbaum et al [24]	965 middle school students	2.7%
Stilger and Yesalis [25]	1325 high school football players	6.3%

Additionally, several national surveys that have not been published or have not been published in their entirety in the peer-review literature, but which have assessed the prevalence of performance-enhancing substance use among United States adolescents, also are presented (Table 3).

Anabolic steroids

Anabolic steroids are synthetic substances that mimic testosterone and are used for increasing fat-free muscle mass and strength, with potentially severe adverse effects. Before their classification as a banned substance with the Anabolic Steroid Control Act of 1990, anabolic steroids were popular performance-enhancing supplements among elite and recreational athletes. These drugs are only available legally by prescription, but they continue to be used illegally by adults and adolescents aiming to gain a physical edge. The prevalence of use depends on several factors and includes participant demographics, such as age, athletic background, and type of sport participation.

Several studies investigated anabolic steroid use among adolescents before and around the time of the implementation of the Anabolic Steroid Control Act of 1990. Buckley and colleagues [18] surveyed male twelfth-grade students from 46 high schools across the country. Results indicated

Table 2
Creatine use among United States adolescents: reports in the peer-review literature

Investigators	Sample population	Overall prevalence
Smith and Dahm [30]	328 high school students	8.2%
Metzl et al [31]	1103 middle/high school athletes	5.6%
Ray et al [32]	674 high school athletes	16.0%
McGuine et al [33]	1349 high school football players	30.0%
McGuine et al [34]	4011 high school athletes	16.7%
Reeder et al [35]	475 high school students	11.0%
Kayton et al [36]	270 high school athletes	13.0%

that 6.6% of the 3403 participants used or had used anabolic steroids. Those who reported use were more likely to participate in sports (67%), the most common of which was football (44%). Reports with similar study populations from around the same time period reported the prevalence of use from 1% to 11% [19–21]. These reports also noted a lack of understanding about the benefits and adverse effects of these substances. Table 1 summarizes peer-review articles reporting anabolic steroid use among adolescents.

Studies that focused on prevalence after the Anabolic Steroid Control Act of 1990 reported a slight decrease in steroid use; however, comparing reports is difficult because of differences in ages and other characteristics. Tanner and colleagues [22] reported overall steroid use of 3% among 6930 high school students in Denver, with boys reporting more use than girls (4% and 1%, respectively). Scott and colleagues [23] reported similar use from their survey of 4722 students from 62 secondary schools; 117 (3%) respondents reported anabolic steroid use in the preceding 30 days, and boys reported use (5%) more than girls (1%). Faigenbaum and colleagues [24] focused on steroid use among 965 middle school students between 9 and 13 years of age. In this population, steroid use was reported by 2.6% of boys and 2.8% of girls, with an overall prevalence of 2.7%. In a survey of 1325 varsity football players from 27 Indiana high schools, Stilger and Yesalis [25] reported the prevalence of use to be 6%.

In addition to the peer-review studies summarized above, three multiyear national surveys have evaluated the prevalence of anabolic steroid use among adolescents (see Table 3) [26–28]. The longest running survey, the Monitoring the Future Study [26], assessed the prevalence of anabolic steroid use among ninth to twelfth graders from 1989 through 2006 in three categories: lifetime use, use over the previous 12 months, and use over the previous 30 days. Because variance in this age group is small, and the prevalence of use is low, only the information for lifetime use by twelfth graders is presented here. This study, which surveyed between 2533 and 7100 twelfth-grade students from across the United States annually, reported prevalence rates of lifetime use of anabolic steroids ranging from a low of 1.9% in 1996 to a high of 4.0% in 2002. The next-longest running survey, the Youth Risk and Behavior Surveillance System [28], evaluated the prevalence of anabolic steroid use among ninth to twelfth graders from 1991 through 2005. This study, which surveyed between 10,904 and 16,262 students from across the United States annually, reported prevalence rates for the lifetime use of anabolic steroids ranging from a low of 2.2% in 1993 to a high of 6.1% in 2003. Across the study period, prevalence rates were consistently higher among boys than among girls, although the gap between genders decreased in 2003 and 2005. The third study, the National Household Survey on Drug Abuse [27], also assessed lifetime use of anabolic steroids. This study, which surveyed between 4678 and 8005 adolescents aged 12 to 17 years from across the United States, only collected information on steroid use from 1991 through 1994. Reported prevalence rates of the lifetime use of anabolic steroids ranged from a low of 0.2% in 1993 to

Table 3
Prevalence of performance-enhancing substance use among United States adolescents: results of national surveys not reported or not fully reported in the peer-review literature

Study	Year	Sample population	Substance	Overall prevalence
Blue Cross and Blue Shield Association's Healthy Competition Foundation National Survey (survey of 10- to 17-year-olds)	2001	785	"Performance-enhancing drugs or sports supplements"	5%
Monitoring the Future Study (survey of 12th graders)	1989	2783	Anabolic steroids (used at least once in lifetime)	3.0%
	1990	2533		2.9%
	1991	5000		2.1%
	1992	5267		2.1%
	1993	5433		2.0%
	1994	5133		2.4%
	1995	5133		2.3%
	1996	4767		1.9%
	1997	5133		2.4%
	1998	5067		2.7%
	1999	4533		2.9%
	2000	4267		2.5%
	2001	4267		3.7%
	2002	4300		4.0%
	2003	4867		3.5%
	2004	4867		3.4%
	2005	4900		2.6%
	2006	7100		2.7%
National Household Survey on Drug Abuse (survey of 12- to 17-year-olds)	1991	8005	Anabolic steroids (used at least once in lifetime)	0.6% (1.0% boys and 0.2% girls)

Survey	Year	Sample	Substance	Prevalence
Youth Athlete Surveys – The Josephson Institute's Report Card Survey Reports (survey of high school athletes)	1992	7254	"Performance-enhancing drugs" (used at least once in past year)	0.3% (0.4% boys and 0.1% girls)
	1993	6978		0.2% (0.3% boys and 0.1% girls)
	1994	4678		0.7% (0.7% boys and 0.6% girls)
	2004	4200		12% boys and 3% girls
	2005 and 2006	5275		6% boys and 2% girls
Youth Risk and Behavior Surveillance System (survey of 9th to 12th graders)	1991	12,272	Anabolic steroids (used at least once in lifetime)	2.7% (4.1% boys and 1.2% girls)
	1993	16,296		2.2% (3.1% boys and 1.2% girls)
	1995	10,904		3.7% (4.9% boys and 2.4% girls)
	1997	16,262		3.1% (4.1% boys and 2.0% girls)
	1999	15,028		3.7% (5.2% boys and 2.2% girls)
	2001	13,627		5.0% (6.0% boys and 3.9% girls)
	2003	15,240		6.1% (6.8% boys and 5.3% girls)
	2005	13,917		4.0% (4.8% boys and 3.2% girls)

a high of 0.6% in 1991. Again, across the study period, prevalence rates were consistently higher among boys than among girls, although the gap was small in 1994. The lower prevalence rates reported in this study compared with the two other national studies likely is due to the broader age range of the sample; published reports consistently have indicated that the use of performance-enhancing substances increases with age throughout adolescence.

The reasons for using anabolic steroids have remained consistent in most studies. Adolescents involved in sports used steroids more often than those who were not, but use was noted among individuals who were not athletes [18,20,23]. Among those who participated in sports activities, use varied by sport. Participating in football was common among users, but so was participation in other sports, such as gymnastics, weight training, basketball, and baseball [18,20,29]. Reasons for using steroids also varied and ranged from improving athletic performance and improving strength among athletes to improving appearance or building self-esteem among those who did not participate in sports activities [18,23,29].

Creatine

Creatine may be the most popular performance-enhancing substance used by adolescents. Creatine is a naturally occurring compound in the body that supplies energy to muscle and is used to enhance recovery after a workout, build muscle mass, and improve strength. There are several recent reports about the prevalence of use of creatine among adolescents (see Table 2).

Smith and Dahm [30] surveyed 328 high school athletes (182 boys and 146 girls) between the ages of 14 and 18 years. Creatine use was reported by 8.2% of boys and 1 girl, use increased with age, and 78% of users were male football players. Additionally, 79% of users reported that creatine improved strength. Most creatine users reported learning about creatine from friends (74%), and most purchased the product from health food stores (89%). Metzl and colleagues [31] surveyed 1103 middle and high school athletes (55% boys, 45% girls) between the ages of 10 and 18 years; 62 (5.6%) respondents reported taking creatine. More boys (8.8%) than girls (1.8%) reported the use of creatine, with use reported by respondents from every grade. Ray and colleagues [32] surveyed 674 athletes from 11 high schools. About 16% of respondents reported using creatine to enhance athletic performance and percentages increased with age. Among those surveyed, 75% had knowledge of creatine supplements.

Two of the largest studies investigating creatine use in adolescents were reported from surveys administered to students in 37 public high schools in Wisconsin [33,34]. McGuine and colleagues [33] reported the results from surveys administered to 1349 high school football players. Creatine use was reported by 10.4% of ninth graders, 23.8% of tenth graders, 41.1% of eleventh graders, and 50.5% of twelfth graders. A subsequent article describing creatine use among 4011 high school athletes reported overall use among 16.7% of respondents (25.3% boys, 3.9% girls). Grade-specific rates included 8.4% of ninth graders, 12.6% of tenth graders, 23.1% of eleventh graders, and 24.6% of twelfth graders [34].

Studies by Reeder and colleagues [35] and Kayton and colleagues [36] evaluated creatine use while investigating a variety of dietary supplements. Reeder and colleagues [35] surveyed 475 high school students and found that creatine was the most popular supplement, with 11.0% of respondents reporting use in the past 12 months. Kayton and colleagues [36] surveyed 270 athletes (55% girls, 45% boys) competing in a winter or spring sport from four different high schools. Creatine use was reported by 13% of students (21% of boys and 3% of girls).

The use of creatine among athletes who participate in different sports is common. Metzl and colleagues [31] reported that the use of creatine varied by sports participation, with a higher percentage of users participating in gymnastics (36%), hockey (20%), wrestling (14.3%), and football (13.4%). McGuine and colleagues [34] reported the distribution of use in sports by gender. Among girls, creatine use was most frequent among athletes who participated in track (5.4%), gymnastics (4.7%), tennis (4.6%), and volleyball (3.8%). Among boys, creatine use was most frequent among athletes who participated in football (30.1%), swimming (28.4%), hockey (28.0%), and baseball (26.5%).

Other performance-enhancing substances

There are many types and formulas of performance-enhancing substances available—legally and illegally—to adolescents today. The prevalence for the use of most performance-enhancing substances among adolescents is largely unknown. A few reports have described the prevalence of use of a few additional types of performance-enhancing substances. Human growth hormone is used to increase muscle mass and strength and has received an increase in media attention and advertising in the past few years; however, little is known about the prevalence of its use as a performance-enhancing supplement. In 1992, Rickert and colleagues [37] reported that use among tenth-grade boys was about 5%.

More recently, Reeder and colleagues [35] surveyed 475 high school students regarding their use of common dietary supplements. Of those surveyed, 20.4% (97 students) reported using at least one supplement in the past 12 months. The most common supplements used were creatine (11.0%), androstenedione (4.0%), and Xenadrine (3%).

Kayton and colleagues [36] surveyed 270 athletes (55% girls, 45% boys) competing in a winter or spring sport from four high schools. Questions about the use of 21 dietary supplements or ergogenic aids were included in the survey. About 22% of respondents reported using dietary supplements to enhance performance, but 58% reported using at least one of the 21 listed dietary supplements for other than ergogenic benefits. Amino acids were used by 8% of boys and 1% of girls, weight gain formula was used by 10% of boys and 2% of girls, and ephedrine was used by 12% of boys and 26% of girls.

General performance-enhancing substance use

Not all reports of the prevalence of performance-enhancing substance use differentiated between the types of such substances. For example, in one national survey [38], high school athletes were asked if they had used "performance-enhancing drugs" in the past year. In this study, there was a much wider range of prevalence of use within genders than between genders, and the reported prevalence was lower in 2005/2006 than in 2004. Although 6% of all male athletes surveyed in 2005/2006 reported the use of performance-enhancing substances, the prevalence of use ranged from a low of 0% among track or volleyball participants to a high of 9%, 10%, and 13% among baseball, hockey, and gymnastics participants, respectively. Similarly, although 2% of all female athletes surveyed in 2005/2006 reported the use of performance-enhancing substances, the prevalence of use ranged from a low of 0% among cross-country, gymnastics, or swimming participants to a high of 3%, 3%, and 4% among cheerleading, softball, and tennis participants, respectively. A national survey of 10- to 17-year-olds [39] reported a prevalence of use of "performance enhancing drugs or sports supplements" of 5%.

Knowledge, attitudes, and beliefs about the use of performance-enhancing substances

Understanding trends over time in the knowledge, attitudes, and beliefs held by adolescent athletes regarding the use of performance-enhancing substances is important to evaluate trends in the prevalence of use in this population and is an essential element of efforts to develop effective preventive interventions. Questions included on national surveys provide insight into this issue. For example, it seems that adolescent athletes may not understand, or at least may not acknowledge, the potential negative health effects of performance-enhancing substances. One national survey [38] indicated that 17% of boys and 10% of girls disagreed with the statement, "No athlete should use performance-enhancing drugs because it's unhealthy." In another national survey [26], when asked how much people risked harming themselves if they took steroids, the percentage of twelfth graders responding that the use of steroids posed "great risk" ranged from a high of 70.7% in 1992 to a low of 55.0% in 2003.

Similarly, adolescent athletes may not hold negative beliefs about the appropriateness of the use of such substances. In one national survey [38], 15% of boys and 11% of girls disagreed with the statement, "No athlete should use performance-enhancing drugs because it's cheating." Also, the proportion of twelfth graders who disapproved of people who took steroids ranged from a high of 92.1% in 1992 to a low of 86.0% in 2003 [26].

Although adolescents seem to have difficulty understanding, or at least acknowledging, the potential negative health effects of performance-enhancing substances and they may fail to attach a negative connotation to the use of such substances, at least one survey indicated that adolescents are knowledgeable about methods of obtaining performance-enhancing substances. In the Monitoring the Future Study [26], from 1991 through 2006, twelfth graders were asked how difficult they believed it would be to get steroids. The proportion of adolescents responding that steroids were "fairly easy" or "very easy" to get remained fairly consistent, ranging from a high of 46.8% in 1992 to a low of 39.7% in 2005.

Summary

Although the reports summarized here demonstrate a wide variance in the prevalence of the use of performance-enhancing substances by gender, age, athlete status, and type of substance, the use of performance-enhancing substances is not uncommon among adolescent athletes who wish to improve their athletic performance as well as among athletic and nonathletic adolescents who wish to improve their appearance. More importantly, there is no evidence to show a consistent decline in the prevalence of the use of performance-enhancing substances in this population. Because adolescents must interpret mixed messages posed by the medical community's opposition to the use of performance enhancing-substances and competing societal rewards for athletic prowess coupled with mass media's body image marketing, there is a clear need for educational information that adolescents will find objective, rational, and readily available.

As eloquently stated by the American Academy of Pediatrics Committee on Sports Medicine and Fitness, pediatricians and other pediatric health care advocates can serve as this much needed "voice of reason" [40]. Pediatric practitioners cannot depend on a passive approach of community education programs or drug testing to curb the use of performance-enhancing substances among adolescents. Rather, pediatric health care providers have an opportunity to fulfill a positive role by gaining knowledge about the recognition and management of performance-enhancing substance use among adolescents and by inquiring about their use during routine health maintenance visits.

References

[1] Emmanquel E. History of pharmacy (Istoria pharmakeutikis). Athens (Greece): Pryssos; 1947. p. 126.
[2] Leder BA, Catlin DH, Longcope C, et al. Metabolism of orally administered androstenedione in young men. J Clin Endocrinol Metab 2001;86:3654–8.
[3] Foley JD, Schydlower M. Anabolic steroid and ergogenic drug use by adolescents. Adolescent Medicine: State of the Art Reviews 1993;4(2):341–53.

[4] Yersalis CE, Courson SP, Wright J. History of anabolic steroid use in sport and exercise. In: Yersalis CE, editor. Anabolic steroids in sport and exercise. Champaign (IL): Human Kinetics; 1993. p. 35–47.

[5] DesJardins M. Supplement use in the adolescent athlete. . Curr Sports Med Rep 2002;1: 369–73.

[6] Glaister M, Lockey RA, Abraham CS, et al. Creatine supplementation and multiple sprint running performance. J Strength Cond Res 2006;20(2):273–7.

[7] Hoffman J, Ratamess N, Kang J, et al. Effect of creatine and beta-alanine supplementation on performance and endocrine responses in strength/power athletes. J Int J Sport Nutr Exerc Metab 2006;16(4):430–46.

[8] Mendes RR, Pires I, Oliveira A, et al. Effects of creatine supplementation on the performance and body composition of competitive swimmers. J Nutr Biochem 2004;15(8): 473–8.

[9] Nissen S, Sharp R, Ray M, et al. Effect of leucine metabolite beta-hydroxy-beta-methylbutyrate on muscle metabolism during resistance exercise training. J Appl Physiol 1996;81(5): 2095–104.

[10] Dietary Supplement Health and Education Act of 1994 (DSHEA). Available at: http://www.cfsan.fda.gov/~;dms/dietsupp.html. Accessed February 28, 2007.

[11] US Anti-Doping Agency. 2007 guide to prohibited substances and prohibited methods of doping. Available at: http://www.usantidoping.org. Accessed February 28, 2007.

[12] Bosworth E, Bents R, Trevesan L, et al. Anabolic steroids and high school athletes. Med Sci Sports Exerc 1987;20(Suppl):3–17.

[13] Hubbell N. The use of steroids by Michigan high school students and athletes: an opinion research study of 10th and 12th grade high school students and varsity athletes, November 1989 through January 1990. Lansing (MI): Department of Public Health, Chronic Disease Advisory Committee; 1990.

[14] Newman M. Michigan Consortium of Schools student survey. Minneapolis (MN): Hazelden Research Services; 1986.

[15] Ringwalt C. Alcohol and other drug use patterns among students in North Carolina public schools, grades 7–12: results of a 1989 student survey. Raleigh (NC): North Carolina Department of Public Instruction, Alcohol and Drug Defense Section, Division of Student Services; 1989.

[16] Ross J, Winters F, Hartmann K, et al. 1988–1989 survey of substance abuse among Maryland adolescents. Baltimore (MD): Department of Health and Mental Hygiene, Alcohol and Drug Abuse Administration; 1989.

[17] vandenBerg P, Neumark-Sztainer D, Cafri G, et al. Steroid use among adolescents: longitudinal findings from Project EAT. Pediatrics 2007;119(3):476–86.

[18] Buckley WE, Yesalis CE 3rd, Friedl KE, et al. Estimated prevalence of anabolic steroid use among male high school seniors. JAMA 1988;260(23):3441–5.

[19] Krowchuk DP, Anglin TM, Goodfellow DB, et al. High school athletes and the use of ergogenic aid. Am J Dis Child 1989;143(4):486–9.

[20] Whitehead R, Chillag S, Elliott D. Anabolic steroid use among adolescents in a rural state. J Fam Pract 1992;35(4):401–5.

[21] Johnson MD, Jay MS, Shoup B, et al. Anabolic steroid use by male adolescents. Pediatrics 1989;83(6):921–4.

[22] Tanner SM, Miller DW, Alongi C. Anabolic steroid use by adolescents: prevalence, motives, and knowledge of risks. Clin J Sport Med 1995;5(2):108–15.

[23] Scott DM, Wagner JC, Barlow TW. Anabolic steroid use among adolescents in Nebraska schools. Am J Health Syst Pharm 1996;53(17):2068–72.

[24] Faigenbaum AD, Zaichkowsky LD, Gardner DE, et al. Anabolic steroid use by male and female middle school students. Pediatrics 1998;101(5):E6.

[25] Stilger VG, Yesalis CE. Anabolic-androgenic steroid use among high school football players. J Community Health 1999;24(2):131–45.

[26] Johnston LD, O'Malley PM, Bachman JG, et al. Monitoring the Future national survey results on drug use, 1975–2006. Available at: http://www.monitoringthefuture.org. Accessed March 15, 2007.

[27] National Household Survey on Drug Abuse. Substance Abuse and Mental Health Services Administration. National Household Survey on Drug Abuse: Population Estimates 1992, 1993, and 1994. Washington, DC: US Dept of Health and Human Services. Publications (ADM) 92-1887, (SMA) 93-2053, (SMA) 94-3017, and (SMA) 95–3063.

[28] Youth Risk and Behavior Surveillance System (YRBSS)—National Center for Chronic Disease Prevention and Health Promotion. Healthy youth! YRBSS, youth online: comprehensive results. General information available at: http://apps.nccd.cdc.gov/yrbss. Information on methodology available at: http://www.cdc.gov/mmwr/PDF/rr/rr5312.pdf. Accessed February 28, 2007.

[29] Radakovich J, Broderick P, Pickell G. Rate of anabolic-androgenic steroid use among students in junior high school. J Am Board Fam Pract 1993;6(4):341–5.

[30] Smith J, Dahm DL. Creatine use among a select population of high school athletes. Mayo Clin Proc 2000;75(12):1257–63.

[31] Metzl JD, Small E, Levine SR, et al. Creatine use among young athletes. Pediatrics 2001; 108(2):421–5.

[32] Ray TR, Eck JC, Covington LA, et al. Use of oral creatine as an ergogenic aid for increased sports performance: perceptions of adolescent athletes. South Med J 2001;94(6):608–12.

[33] McGuine TA, Sullivan JC, Bernhardt DT. Creatine supplementation in high school football players. Clin J Sport Med 2001;11(4):247–53.

[34] McGuine TA, Sullivan JC, Bernhardt DA. Creatine supplementation in Wisconsin high school athletes. WMJ 2002;101(2):25–30.

[35] Reeder BM, Rai A, Patel DR, et al. The prevalence of nutritional supplement use among high school students: a pilot study. Med Sci Sports Exerc 2002;34(5):S193.

[36] Kayton S, Cullen RW, Memken JA, et al. Supplement and ergogenic aid use by competitive male and female high school athletes. Med Sci Sports Exerc 2002;34(5):S193.

[37] Rickert VI, Pawlak-Morello C, Sheppard V, et al. Human growth hormone: a new substance of abuse among adolescents? Clin Pediatr 1992;31(12):723–6.

[38] Youth athlete survey—The Josephson Institute's Report Card Survey Reports. Available at: http://www.josephsoninstitute.org/sports_survey/2006/. Accessed February 22, 2007.

[39] Blue Cross and Blue Shield Association's Healthy Competition Foundation National Survey on PEDs in Sports Summary of Key Survey Results, 2001. Power point presentation available at: http://ods.od.nih.gov/news/conferences/ShaferScience_and_Policy.pdf. Summary result release available at: http://64.233.167.104/search?q=cache:7esxIdqQa5EJ: www.healthycompetition.org/hc/news/supplement_survey.html+Survey+projects+1+million+ youths+aged+12-17+use+potentially+dangerous+sports+supplements+and+drugs&;hl= en&ct=clnk&cd=1&gl=us. Accessed February 28, 2007.

[40] American Academy of Pediatrics Committee on Sports Medicine and Fitness. Adolescents and anabolic steroids: a subject review. Pediatrics 1997;99:904–8.

ELSEVIER
SAUNDERS

PEDIATRIC CLINICS
OF NORTH AMERICA

Pediatr Clin N Am 54 (2007) 677–690

Consequences of Use of Anabolic Androgenic Steroids

Marcel J. Casavant, MD[a,b,c],*, Kathleen Blake, MD[a],
Jill Griffith, PharmD[c,d], Andrew Yates, MD[a,e],
LaRae M. Copley, RPh, MD, PhD[a,f]

[a]*Department of Pediatrics, The Ohio State University College of Medicine,
370 West 9th Ave., Columbus, OH 43210, USA*
[b]*Department of Emergency Medicine, The Ohio State University College of Medicine,
1654 Upham Drive Columbus, OH 43210, USA*
[c]*Central Ohio Poison Center at Children's Hospital, 700 Children's Drive,
Columbus, OH 43205, USA*
[d]*The Ohio State University College of Pharmacy, 500 West 12th Ave., Columbus,
OH 43210, USA*
[e]*Division of Cardiology, Children's Hospital, 700 Children's Drive,
Columbus, OH 43205, USA*
[f]*Department of Psychiatry, The Ohio State University Hospitals, 140 Neurosciences Facility,
1670 Upham Drive, Columbus, OH 43210, USA*

Whether providing anticipatory guidance to the young adolescent patient, conducting a preparticipation examination on a young athlete, or treating a sick user of anabolic androgenic steroids (AASs), the primary care physician must be familiar with the adverse consequences of the use of these compounds. This article reviews the endocrine, cardiovascular, neuropsychiatric, musculoskeletal, hematologic, hepatic, and miscellaneous effects of AASs, highlighting effects reported in children and adolescents and relying on consequences in adults when pediatric data are unavailable. We rely heavily on case reports and series; prospective studies are rare for technical and ethical reasons and are of questionable generalizability, given the number of AASs and the variety of dose ranges and patterns of use. The available data may underestimate the actual untoward effects because doses

* Corresponding author. Central Ohio Poison Center at Children's Hospital, 700 Children's Drive, E-265, Columbus, OH 43205.
E-mail address: casavant@chi.osu.edu (M.J. Casavant).

0031-3955/07/$ - see front matter © 2007 Elsevier Inc. All rights reserved.
doi:10.1016/j.pcl.2007.04.001
pediatric.theclinics.com

administered in clinical studies do not approximate the supraphysiologic doses used by illicit steroid users.

Endocrine consequences

The adverse endocrine effects of AASs are best understood if one first looks at the native effects of testosterone. Testosterone is responsible for the in utero masculinization of internal genitalia, postnatal skeletal muscle development, and the development of male secondary sexual characteristics. In addition, testosterone is converted in peripheral tissues by 5-alpha-reductase to dihydrotestosterone (DHT), which contributes to fetal development of external genitalia, prostate, and seminal vesicles. DHT acts in the cell nucleus of target tissues, such as skin, male accessory glands, and the prostate, exerting predominantly androgenic, but also anabolic, effects. Testosterone is converted by the enzyme aromatase to estradiol and estrone, which are involved in the sexual differentiation of the brain, bone mass accretion, and fusion of the epiphyses at the conclusion of puberty, in addition to feminizing effects [1]. Under normal physiologic circumstances, aromatase has a limited role; however, with high-dose AAS use, this role increases, and, therefore, so does the level of estrogens [2]. An antiestrogen effect may be present as well with supraphysiologic doses of AASs. Excess AASs lead to a down-regulation of androgen receptors and AASs then compete with estrogens for the estrogen receptor. The net outcome of these two different pathways is difficult to predict [3]. With this information, it is easier to understand the adverse outcomes of AAS use because many of the effects are amplifications of physiologic effects.

Testosterone acts at the androgen receptor to increase protein synthesis; it also has effects through conversion to DHT and estrogens. At normal physiologic levels of testosterone, androgen receptors are saturated, and it is believed that some of the effects of AASs may be through one or more different mechanisms. Research has shown an antagonist effect at the glucocorticoid receptor at supraphysiologic levels that leads to an anticatabolic effect [4]. Glucocorticoids influence glucose synthesis and protein catabolism. The stimulation of glucocorticoid receptors by glucocorticoids leads to increased protein breakdown in muscle. High-dose AASs may displace glucocorticoids from the glucocorticoid receptor and inhibit muscle protein breakdown that leads to an overall anabolic or muscle-building effect [5]. By competing with glucocorticoids for the glucocorticoid receptor, AASs block the depressed protein synthesis that usually occurs during stressful training. AASs also exert some effect on the growth hormone (GH)–insulin-like growth factor (IGF)-1 axis. There seems to be an androgen-induced stimulation of GH secretion and a direct stimulation of hepatic IGF-1 synthesis. IGF-1 stimulates skeletal muscle formation, and GH exhibits anabolic effects [6,7]. AASs act on osteoblasts to stimulate proliferation and differentiation that may inhibit bone breakdown. There also may be some degree of "placebo effect" that allows AAS users to train harder and increase muscle mass as a result of the increased aggression, euphoria, and decreased fatigue and recovery time that many AAS users report [2,4].

In men, chronic AAS use can lead to decreased endogenous testosterone production and hypogonadotropic hypogonadism associated with testicular atrophy. Chronic AAS abuse causes a decrease in gonadotropins, luteinizing hormone (LH), and follicle-stimulating hormone (FSH) as part of the negative feedback system of the hypothalamic-pituitary-gonadal axis. LH and FSH are needed for spermatogenesis so when these hormones are decreased, there is a decrease in sperm count and mobility as well as an increase in the number of morphologically abnormal sperm [2,3,8–10]. One study found a 73% overall decrease in sperm count; three individuals had azoospermia with chronic use of high-dose AASs. In individuals who did not experience azoospermia, there was a 10% increase in the number of immotile sperm and a 30% decrease in the number of motile sperm. Overall, fertility was severely reduced [11]. Decreases in gonadotropins can be seen within 24 hours of beginning AASs. Infertility may result within months [2]. After cessation of use, gonadotropin and testosterone secretion are suppressed for months to years. Usually, the infertility is spontaneously reversible, typically within 1 year of cessation of AAS abuse, but it may take longer in long-term users [10]. At least one user of multiple AASs did not recover fertility spontaneously and required treatment with LH-releasing hormone to regain normal levels of testosterone and fertility [12]. Men also may experience priapism, impotence, prostatic hypertrophy, difficulty/pain with urination, and a possible increased risk for prostate cancer [13]. The risk for these consequences increases with dose and duration of use [6].

Testosterone is converted to estrogens by aromatase and to DHT by way of 5-alpha reductase. The estrogens lead to feminizing effects in men, such as gynecomastia and an increase in voice pitch. Although the breast tissue that develops becomes softer and less prominent after cessation of AAS use, this effect may be irreversible and require surgical correction [8,10]. Men experience male-pattern baldness, acne (mostly on the trunk), and altered libido [9], which likely is due to the effects of DHT. Acne is the result of androgenic stimulation of sebaceous glands [1].

The sexual and reproductive effects of AAS are more dramatic in women [14]. Although AASs have been developed to try to minimize androgen effects, all AASs exert some degree of virilizing effects if given for long enough and in sufficiently large doses. Virilization occurs with AAS use by women, regardless of the type used. Early effects include acne, deepening of the voice, and changes in libido. Deepening of the voice occurs as a result of laryngeal hypertrophy. Long-term use can lead to clitoral enlargement, male-pattern baldness, and alterations in pubic hair. Other virilizing effects include decreased body fat, breast atrophy, amenorrhea or oligomenorrhea, uterine atrophy, and hirsutism [1,13]. The changes in menses are due to suppression of the hypothalamic-pituitary-gonadal axis [1]. Some of these effects may be irreversible with chronic use [1,2,6,9,10,13,15]. AASs may act as a teratogen [13].

Children seem to be the most susceptible to the adverse effects of AAS use [15]. Children and adolescents experience accelerated maturation associated with changes in physique and earlier development of secondary sexual characteristics [13]. An additional concern with adolescents is premature closure of growth plates in long bones, leading to a decrease in final height; this likely is due to aromatization to estrogens [1,2,9]. Precocious puberty in boys and contrasexual precocity in girls also can occur [15]. With adolescents, some of the effects may become irreversible with chronic use, particularly the virilizing effects in young women [6,14,15].

Thyroid cells have androgen receptors, and AASs may directly influence thyroid function [16]. Some studies have shown effects on thyroid function, including a decrease in total triiodothyronine, thyroxine (T_4), and thyroid-binding globulin. Some studies have shown an increase in thyrotropin and free T_4, whereas others have shown no change in these concentrations. It is unclear if this relative impairment in thyroid function leads to a clinical effect. These changes may be due to direct block of thyroid hormone release or synthesis or some other mechanism [16–18]. AASs decrease glucose tolerance and increase insulin resistance, which lead to hyperinsulinism and secondary diabetes mellitus with type II symptoms [2,3,9,11,13].

Many AAS users take additional drugs or supplements to counteract the adverse effects of AASs [19]. Among 500 users of AASs, more than 50% reported taking clomiphene, antiaromatases (eg, anastrozole), or the antiestrogen tamoxifen; 40% admitted to using human chorionic gonadotropin [4]. Human chorionic gonadotropin and clomiphene are taken at the end of or after an AAS cycle to reduce hypogonadotropic hypogonadism and reverse testicular atrophy and infertility. Some studies have shown maintenance of spermatogenesis with the concurrent use of human chorionic gonadotropin, but there are still significantly more abnormal and hypokinetic spermatozoa. The maintenance of spermatogenesis by human chorionic gonadotropin occurs without an increase in FSH. The low FSH concentration explains why sperm quality remains abnormal [4]. The effect on offspring is unknown [20]. The side effects of human chorionic gonadotropin include hyperglycemia, insulin resistance, decreased thyroid function, adrenal insufficiency, carpal tunnel syndrome, arthralgia, myopathy, pancreatitis, hepatotoxicity, and an increased risk for certain malignancies [21]. Clomiphene stimulates the release of gonadotropins and is used in women with infertility; however, clomiphene may not increase serum gonadotropins when taken by power athletes during an AAS cycle [20]. Antiaromatase or antiestrogen drugs, such as anastrozole and tamoxifen, are taken to counteract the effects of aromatization of the AAS to estrogens (eg, gynecomastia). There is no data to support their effectiveness, and they also have side effects [2].

Cardiovascular consequences

The most common cardiovascular consequences of AAS include athero-sclerosis (secondary to changes in cholesterol metabolism and platelet function), hypertension, cardiac hypertrophy, impaired cardiac function, and sudden death [22–24].

AAS use causes metabolic derangements that increase the risk for athero-sclerosis and thrombus formation. Studies using animal models and various steroid regimens have demonstrated changes in serum cholesterol levels with decreased high-density lipoprotein and increased low-density lipoprotein, both promoting atherosclerotic and peripheral vascular disease [2,25,26]. Cholesterol alterations vary among different AASs; alkylated agents (eg, stanozolol) cause greater changes than testosterone [27].

AAS use also increases platelet reactivity without an associated thrombo-cytosis; this has been proposed as an etiology for some of the myocardial infarctions, strokes, and peripheral vascular disease events reported in otherwise healthy individuals [28,29]. AAS use also increases serum C-reactive protein (CRP), reflecting an inflammatory state that may contribute to atheroma formation and peripheral vascular disease [30]. Conversely, changes in lipid metabolism may be protective from atheroma formation because of a reduction in lipoprotein A [25]. Many studies show that AASs cause abnormal cholesterol profiles, increased CRP, and increased platelet reactivity. It is difficult to quantify the change in risk, but one study estimates AASs triple the cardiovascular risk [31].

Systemic hypertension is a side effect of medical steroid administration and may require antihypertensive therapy; therefore, high-dose ASA use also should result in systemic hypertension. This is found in some reports [23,32], but not consistently [33]. AAS-induced hypertension may be related to vascular endothelial response [34], increased responsiveness to catechol-amines [35], and increased renin production [36]. The magnitude and inci-dence of hypertension likely are related to dosage and to the specific AAS.

Recent echocardiographic studies of AAS users demonstrate an increase in septal and left ventricular posterior wall thickness. This hypertrophy is greater in weight-trained individuals using AASs than in weight-trained individuals provided placebo or not using AASs [34,37–41] and persists for years among former AAS users [40]. Cardiac wall hypertrophy may not occur after short-term ASA use [26,42,43].

AAS use impairs measures of diastolic function (eg, isovolumetric relax-ation time [37] and altered tissue Doppler imaging of the left ventricle [44,45]) that reflect impaired relaxation and altered filling during diastole. Possible etiologies for impaired diastolic function include increased collagen content [46] or areas of focal necrosis, seen at autopsy of AAS users [47,48].

Cardiovascular performance also can be assessed by way of formal exer-cise testing; although AASs may increase bulk and strength, they do not im-prove endurance. Despite having similar aerobic and weight-training schedules as control subjects, AAS users had a significantly decreased maximum oxygen consumption (Vo_2max; an index of metabolic and cardiovascular endurance ability) [38]. Impaired diastolic function could contribute to decreased Vo_2max.

Sudden death is the most frightening consequence of AAS use. The etiology of these events likely is multifactorial, with AAS use contributing to the observed pathology. There are case reports of myocardial infarctions [49], stroke, and peripheral vascular obstruction [50] from thrombus that likely are related to the changes in platelet function, inflammation, and cholesterol metabolism discussed above. Autopsies of 34 users of AASs found chronic cardiac changes consisting of cardiac hypertrophy, myocardial fibrosis, and coronary artery atheromatous changes in 12 victims, although these were believed to contribute to the deaths of only 2 victims [48].

Many sudden death events among AAS users have been due to ischemia secondary to coronary artery disease; however, there is a report of ventricular tachycardia during exercise testing of an AAS user who had myocardial fibrosis on biopsy [51]. Other case reports of sudden death demonstrate diffuse, patchy fibrotic changes in the myocardium of AAS users without coronary artery atherosclerosis [47]. The presence of scar or infiltrative processes is commonly believed to be a cause for arrhythmia. The exact cause of sudden death in AAS users is unclear but likely is due to ischemia or arrhythmia.

Neurologic and psychiatric consequences

In a recent study in middle and high school students, 5.4% of boys and 2.9% of girls had used steroids in the previous year [52]. Use in boys was associated with higher rates of depressed mood, prior suicide attempts, greater substance abuse, and lower self-esteem. Another study of adolescents suggested that steroid use was associated with other high-risk behaviors and was less likely to be an isolated behavior [53]. Although pediatric data are scarce, psychiatric, behavioral, and neurologic consequences of AAS use are well described [54–58].

Many case reports describe psychiatric symptoms in patients using AASs [48,59–63]. Reports of suicide include at least one patient who did not have a personal or family history of depression or suicidal behaviors [59]. In one series of eight suicides in AAS users from Sweden, collateral information was sought, and when possible, psychologic autopsies were performed [60]. Retrospectively, psychiatric symptoms, such as irritability, aggressiveness ("roid rage"), mood swings, decreased impulse control, and increased energy were noted during AAS use; however, the series included men who had prior psychiatric syndromes, personality disorders, and other substance abuse. Another report showed homicidal or near homicidal behavior in three men during AAS use [61]. None had a history of psychiatric illness or violence before AAS use, and all met the *Diagnostic and Statistical*

Manual of Mental Disorders, Revised Third Edition criteria for manic epi-
sode during use. Two of the three men experienced depression and suicidal
ideation upon the abrupt discontinuation of use. Although it is tempting to
attribute this behavior to AAS use, this is a small set of case studies and as
the investigators note, legal ramifications for the patients may have led to
exaggeration in their reports. A series of 34 deaths of AAS users revealed
nine victims of homicide, 11 suicides, 12 accidental deaths, and 2 deaths
of indeterminate cause [48]. The homicide victims showed high levels of
aggression; in most of the suicide and accidental deaths, impulsive and violent behaviors had been noted by family or physicians. Most of the cases
of accidental death were related to polysubstance overdose; four of the victims were heroin addicts who had histories of only sporadic or moderate
AAS use.

One study identified seven AAS users and evaluated them every 2 weeks for
as long as 44 weeks [62]. During clinic visits, subjects reported their AAS use,
and assessments, including the Beck Depression Inventory (BDI), Profile of
Mood States Questionnaire, and Buss-Durkee Hostility Scale, were administered. Scores fluctuated over time, but the fluctuations were not associated
with AAS use. Additionally, most of the subjects had a history of major depression, and five reported abusing other substances. A larger study (n = 160)
comparing AAS-using athletes with nonusing athletes revealed that far more
AAS users displayed mood disorders compared with nonusers and AAS users
during periods of no use [64]. Another study describing 41 AAS-using athletes
reported that 22% displayed mood syndromes during use, which was significantly higher than the rate observed during periods of no exposure [65]. Additionally, this study reported that 12.2% displayed psychotic symptoms
during use compared with 0% during AAS-free periods. Another naturalistic
study comparing weight-lifting AAS users with nonusers correlated supranor-
mal testosterone levels with subjective and objective measures of aggression
[66]. Cluster B personality traits, including antisocial, borderline, and histri-
onic, were more prominent in AAS users.

Attempts have been made to study the effects of AASs in humans in
prospective laboratory-controlled settings. One double-blind study administered placebo followed by low-dose (40 mg/d) and then high-dose (240 mg/d)
methyltestosterone to 20 normal healthy men without psychiatric disease
or history of AAS use [67]. During the high-dose period (3 days), distractibility, irritability, and energy level increased significantly, and there was
a trend for an increase in anger and violent feelings. One subject developed
acute mania, and another developed hypomania. Subtle, but significant,
elevations in the BDI, Hamilton Depression Rating Scale, Brief Psychiatric
Rating Scale, and hostility, anxiety and somatization on the Symptom
Checklist (SCL-90) were observed. In follow-up studies, an increase in
aggressiveness correlated with an increase in free T_4, an increase in forget-
fulness and distractibility correlated with total testosterone levels, and an
increase in activation symptoms (energy, sexual arousal, and diminished

sleep) correlated with cerebrospinal fluid 5-hydroxyindole acetic acid levels [18,68]. In another placebo-controlled cross-over study of 50 men free of substance abuse or psychiatric illness, increasing levels of testosterone cypionate were administered over 6 weeks [69]. Aggressive responses on the Point Subtraction Aggression Paradigm and increased manic scores on the Young Mania Rating Scale were demonstrated; 84% showed minimal psychiatric symptoms, 12% became mildly hypomanic, and 4% became markedly hypomanic. An additional study evaluated testosterone cypionate over 14 weeks at levels up to 500 mg/wk in healthy men free of psychiatric illnesses and personality disorders; it found minimal psychologic effects in most men, but one adverse psychiatric effect resembled mania [70]. Additionally, some studies showed no changes in psychometric measures in healthy men who were administered AASs [71]. All of these studies used doses lower than those typical in AAS use, so they likely underestimated the psychiatric consequences of AAS.

Musculoskeletal consequences

Muscle mass seems to be affected greatly by AAS dosing. Higher doses have been shown to garner increases in muscle mass [2]. Muscle mass gains are larger when AAS use is combined with strength training compared with AAS use alone. AASs increase the number of myonuclei. Strenuous exercise seems to increase the number of androgen receptor sites on the muscle. Body weight increases can be in the range of 2 to 5 kg after 10 weeks of AAS use. With more androgen receptors present in the upper regions of the body, the neck, shoulders, thorax, and upper arms gain the most new bulk [2]. The thigh muscles require higher doses to show measurable increases in mass and are not as likely to show increases in the number of androgen receptors [72,73]. Upon discontinuation, muscles shrink and strength declines over a period of 6 to 12 weeks.

Androgens stimulate osteoblast proliferation and differentiation and inhibit the osteoclast. At the start of puberty, androgens stimulate bone formation. At the end of puberty, they induce epiphyseal closure. In adulthood, the sex hormones slow the rate of bone remodeling, protect against bone loss, encourage bone formation, and increase bone density [2].

The adolescent AAS user risks an increased rate of muscle strains or ruptures [3,74]. Unlike muscles, tendons do not increase in strength so with more intense training, they have a greater risk for rupture [75–77]. In a developing adolescent, the growth plate cartilage is considered the "weakest link," and generally is more prone to injury compared with ligaments [78]. A rapid increase in the intensity, frequency, or volume of training is noted consistently in athletes who present with overuse injuries. Injury to the growth plate from weight training has long been a subject of controversy; power lifting may increase the risk for injury, even in adolescents not taking AASs [79,80]. Of particular concern in this age group is premature physeal closure resulting in decreased adult height [3].

AAS users also are at risk for rhabdomyolysis or acute skeletal muscle destruction. Rhabdomyolysis has been reported after vigorous weight lifting and may be more likely in patients escalating and supplementing weight training with AASs [81,82]. Physicians should consider the creatine phosphokinase and gamma-glutamyl transpeptidase levels as essential elements in distinguishing muscle damage from liver damage when evaluating enzyme elevations in patients who use anabolic steroids [83].

Hematologic consequences

Before the introduction of recombinant human erythropoietin, AASs were used in the treatment of anemias. AASs increase renal synthesis of erythropoietin. They also promote erythropoietic stem cell differentiation. Subsequently, hemoglobin and hematocrit may become elevated, which could result in erythrocytosis or sludging [13].

Two adult cases of intramuscular testosterone–induced polycythemia were reportedly reversed by switching to transdermal testosterone [84]; however a 65-year-old man developed hypertension and polycythemia during daily testosterone application to his scrotum for 5 years (estimated dose 10 mg/d). Polycythemia and hypertension resolved when testosterone was discontinued [85].

Mild, but significant, increases in mean red blood cell, hematocrit, hemoglobin, and white blood cell concentrations in 33 men were reported following intramuscular testosterone enanthate, 200 mg every 3 or four weeks for 24 weeks [86]. The men remained asymptomatic.

Increased platelet count and aggregation also may occur. AASs may potentiate platelet aggregation and be thrombogenic in humans [30,87]; however, another study found only nonsignificant trends, including thrombocytosis and increased aggregation [28].

Suppression of clotting factors II, V, VII, and X and bleeding in patients receiving concomitant anticoagulant therapy have been reported with testosterone [88,89]. Case reports demonstrated that coadministration of oral anticoagulants and 17-alkylated androgens (fluoxymesterone, oxandrolone, oxymetholone, methyltestosterone, methandrostenolone, stanozolol) resulted in a prolonged prothrombin time and hemorrhages; AASs may reduce the need for therapeutic anticoagulants by 25% [90].

Hepatic consequences

Multiple hepatic consequences of AAS use are reported, ranging from benign and reversible to permanent and life threatening. None is universal; the incidence of each may vary with dosage, length of use, and specific AAS chosen; alkylated AASs are particularly hepatotoxic [27]. Cholestasis is common, but often is asymptomatic or associated with subclinical elevation of hepatic transaminases [91]. Hepatocellular hyperplasia and elevations of transaminases, conjugated bilirubin, alkaline phosphatase, and lactate dehydrogenase occur [27]. Early elevation of transaminases without increasing gamma-glutamyl transpeptidase may represent muscle damage; serum creatine phosphokinase should be measured [2]. Dose-dependent jaundice is common after several months of AAS use and usually resolves after discontinuing AAS use [10]. Steroid "cycling" is believed to reduce cholestasis and jaundice. Benign hepatic adenomas and rarer hepatocellular carcinoma have been reported in association with AAS use [2,3,10,27]. Regression of adenomas after avoidance of AAS has occurred; death from carcinoma also has occurred [27,91]. Peliosis hepatis is the presence of blood-filled cavities in the liver; this has occurred with iatrogenic AAS use and with AAS abuse. Sometimes reversible, peliosis hepatis can cause liver failure, and the rupture of these cysts can cause fatal internal hemorrhage [15,27,91].

Miscellaneous consequences

Acutely, injections of AAS may lead to bacterial or viral infections from use of contaminated needles or lack of sterile technique. Of concern with deep intramuscular administration are local tissue reactions to the oil diluent, cellulitis, as well as bacterial and fungal abscesses. These infections are related primarily to nonsterile injection technique and shared injection equipment; they are avoidable [92]. Other skin findings may include increased keloid formation and injection track marks.

Users of high-dose AAS regimens report a withdrawal syndrome, including steroid craving, depression, suicidality, irritability, muscle aches, and autonomic instability including hot flashes, nausea and vomiting, tachycardia, and hypertension [3,27].

Adolescent users could be susceptible to all of the above adverse effects. There exists a great division between the conviction of athletes that AASs are effective and the conviction of clinicians that they are harmful. Rather than teaching that these products are ineffective, which will only convince the patient of the clinician's unreliability, it may be more prudent first to acknowledge the common increase in muscle mass that accompanies AAS use, and then to teach about the common, manageable, and minor side effects and the more severe, often irreversible, unpredictable toxicities. It is hoped that coaches, trainers, and clinicians share the same goal of a drug-free sports experience for young athletes; showing role models who achieve their physical goals without AAS use can be helpful in providing realistic alternatives to drug use [3].

References

[1] Wu FCW. Endocrine aspects of anabolic steroids. Clin Chem 1997;43(7):1289–92.

[2] Hartgnes F, Kuipers H. Effects of androgenic-anabolic steroids in athletes. Sports Med 2004; 34(8):513–54.

[3] American Academy of Pediatrics, Committee on Sports Medicine and Fitness. Adolescents and anabolic steroids: a subject review. Pediatrics 1997;99(6):904–8.

[4] Parkinson AB, Evans NA. Anabolic androgenic steroids: a survey of 500 users. Med Sci Sports Exerc 2006;38(4):644–51.

[5] Mottram DR, George AJ. Anabolic steroids. Baillieres Best Pract Res Clin Endocrinol Metab 2000;14(1):55–69.

[6] Evans NA. Current concepts in anabolic-androgenic steroids. Am J Sports Med 2004;32(2): 534–42.

[7] Kuhn CM. Anabolic steroids. Recent Prog Horm Res 2002;57:411–34.

[8] Ciocca M. Medication and supplement use by athletes. Clin Sports Med 2005;24:719–38.

[9] Parssinen M, Seppala T. Steroid use and long-term health risks in former athletes. Sports Med 2002;32(2):83–94.

[10] Brown JT. Anabolic steroids: what should the emergency physician know? Emerg Med Clin North Am 2005;23:815–26.

[11] Holma PK. Effects of anabolic steroid (metandienone) on spermatogenesis. Contraception 1977;15(2):151–62.

[12] Van Breda E, Keizer HA, Kuipers H, et al. Androgenic anabolic steroid use and severe hypothalamic-pituitary dysfunction: a case study. Int J Sports Med 2003;24:195–6.

[13] Maravelias C, Dona A, Stefanidou M, et al. Adverse effects of anabolic steroids in athletes: a constant threat. Toxicol Lett 2005;158:167–75.

[14] Clark AS, Costine BA, Jones BL, et al. Sex- and age-specific effects of anabolic androgenic steroids on reproductive behaviors and on GABAergic transmission in neuroendocrine control regions. Brain Res 2006;1126(1):122–38.

[15] Chyka PA. Androgenic-anabolic steroids. In: Ford MD, editor. Clinical toxicology. 1st edition. Philadelphia: WB Saunders; 2001. p. 595–600.

[16] Fortunato FS, Marassi MP, Chaves EA, et al. Chronic administration of anabolic androgenic steroid alters murine thyroid function. Med Sci in Sports Exerc 2006;38(2): 256–61.

[17] Deyssig R, Weissel M. Ingestions of androgenic-anabolic steroids induces mild thyroidal impairment in male body builders. J Clin Endocrinol Metab 1993;76(4):1069–71.

[18] Daly RC, Su TP, Schmidt PJ, et al. Neuroendocrine and behavioral effects of high-dose anabolic steroid administration in male normal volunteers. Psychoneuroendocrinology 2003;28:317–31.

[19] Brower KJ. Anabolic steroid abuse and dependence. Curr Psychiatry Rep 2002;4:377–87.

[20] Karila T, Hovatta O, Seppala T. Concomitant abuse of anabolic androgenic steroids and human chorionic gonadotropin impairs spermatogenesis in power athletes. Int J Sports Med 2004;25:257–63.

[21] Patel DR, Greydanus DE, Luckstead EF. The college athlete. Pediatr Clin North Am 2005; 52:25–60.

[22] Thiblin I, Petersson A. Pharmacoepidemiology of anabolic androgenic steroids: a review. Fundam Clin Pharmacol 2005;19(1):27–44.

[23] Sullivan ML, Martinez CM, Gennes P, et al. The cardiac toxicity of anabolic steroids. Prog Cardiovasc Dis 1998;41(1):1–15.

[24] Dhar R, Stout CW, Link MS, et al. Cardiovascular toxicities of performance-enhancing substances in sports. Mayo Clin Proc 2005;80(10):1307–15.

[25] Cohen LI, Hartford CG, Rogers GG. Lipoprotein (a) and cholesterol in body builders using anabolic androgenic steroids. Med Sci Sports Exerc 1996;28(2):176–9.

[26] Palatini P, Giada F, Garavelli G, et al. Cardiovascular effects of anabolic steroids in weight-trained subjects. J Clin Pharmacol 1996;36(12):1132–40.

[27] Hall RCW, Hall RCW. Abuse of supraphysiologic doses of anabolic steroids. South Med J 2005;98:550–5.

[28] Ferenchick G, Schwartz D, Ball M. Androgenic-anabolic steroid abuse and platelet aggregation: a pilot study in weight lifters. Am J Med Sci 1992;303(2):78–82.

[29] Ferenchick GS. Anabolic/androgenic steroid abuse and thrombosis: is there a connection? Med Hypotheses 1991;35(1):27–31.

[30] Grace FM, Davies B. Raised concentrations of C reactive protein in anabolic steroid using bodybuilders. Br J Sports Med 2004;38(1):97–8.

[31] Glazer G. Atherogenic effects of anabolic steroids on serum lipid levels. A literature review. Arch Intern Med 1991;151(10):1925–33.

[32] Lenders JW, Demacker PN, Vos JA, et al. Deleterious effects of anabolic steroids on serum lipoproteins, blood pressure, and liver function in amateur body builders. Int J Sports Med 1988;9(1):19–23.

[33] Kuipers H, Wijnen JA, Hartgens F, et al. Influence of anabolic steroids on body composition, blood pressure, lipid profile and liver functions in body builders. Int J Sports Med 1991;12(4):413–8.

[34] Sader MA, Griffiths KA, McCredie RJ, et al. Androgenic anabolic steroids and arterial structure and function in male bodybuilders. J Am Coll Cardiol 2001;37(1):224–30.

[35] Greenberg S, George WR, Kadowitz PJ, et al. Androgen-induced enhancement of vascular reactivity. Can J Physiol Pharmacol 1974;52(1):14–22.

[36] Katz FH, Roper EF. Testosterone effect on renin system in rats. Proc Soc Exp Biol Med 1977;155(3):330–3.

[37] De Piccoli B, Giada F, Benettin A, et al. Anabolic steroid use in body builders: an echocardiographic study of left ventricle morphology and function. Int J Sports Med 1991;12(4):408–12.

[38] Sachtleben TR, Berg KE, Elias BA, et al. The effects of anabolic steroids on myocardial structure and cardiovascular fitness. Med Sci Sports Exerc 1993;25(11):1240–5.

[39] Karila TA, Karjalainen JE, Mantysaari MJ, et al. Anabolic androgenic steroids produce dose-dependant increase in left ventricular mass in power athletes, and this effect is potentiated by concomitant use of growth hormone. Int J Sports Med 2003;24(5):337–43.

[40] Urhausen A, Albers T, Kindermann W. Are the cardiac effects of anabolic steroid abuse in strength athletes reversible? Heart 2004;90(5):496–501.

[41] Dickerman RD, Schaller F, McConathy WJ. Left ventricular wall thickening does occur in elite power athletes with or without anabolic steroid use. Cardiology 1998;90(2):145–8.

[42] Thompson PD, Sadaniantz A, Cullinane EM, et al. Left ventricular function is not impaired in weight-lifters who use anabolic steroids. J Am Coll Cardiol 1992;19(2):278–82.

[43] Hartgens F, Cheriex EC, Kuipers H. Prospective echocardiographic assessment of androgenic-anabolic steroids effects on cardiac structure and function in strength athletes. Int J Sports Med 2003;24(5):344–51.

[44] Nottin S, Nguyen L, Terbah M, et al. Cardiovascular effects of androgenic anabolic steroids in male bodybuilders determined by tissue Doppler imaging. Am J Cardiol 2006;97(6):912–5.

[45] Kindermann W, Urhausen A. Left ventricular dimensions and function in strength athletes. Re: Hartgens F, Cheriex EC, Kuipers H. Prospective echocardiographic assessment of androgenic-anabolic steroids effects on cardiac structure and function in strength athletes. Int J Sports Med 2003;24:344–51. Int J Sports Med 2004;25(3):241–2 [author reply: 243–4].

[46] Di Bello V, Giorgi D, Bianchi M, et al. Effects of anabolic-androgenic steroids on weightlifters' myocardium: an ultrasonic videodensitometric study. Med Sci Sports Exerc 1999;31(4):514–21.

[47] Luke JL, Farb A, Virmani R, et al. Sudden cardiac death during exercise in a weight lifter using anabolic androgenic steroids: pathological and toxicological findings. J Forensic Sci 1990;35(6):1441–7.

[48] Thiblin I, Lindquist O, Rajs J. Cause and manner of death among users of anabolic androgenic steroids. J Forensic Sci 2000;45(1):16–23.

[49] Halvorsen S, Thorsby PM, Haug E. [Acute myocardial infarction in a young man who had been using androgenic anabolic steroids]. Tidsskr Nor Laegeforen 2004;124(2):170–2 [in Norwegian].

[50] Laroche GP. Steroid anabolic drugs and arterial complications in an athlete–a case history. Angiology 1990;41(11):964–9.

[51] Nieminen MS, Rämö M, Viitasalo P, et al. Serious cardiovascular side effects of large doses of anabolic steroids in weight lifters. Eur Heart J 1996;17(10):1576–83.

[52] Irving LM, Wall M, Neumark-Sztainer D, et al. Steroid use among adolescents: findings from Project EAT. J Adolesc Health 2002;30:243–52.

[53] Middleman AB, Faulkner AH, Woods ER, et al. High-risk behaviors among high school students in Massachusetts who use anabolic steroids. Pediatrics 1995;96:268–72.

[54] Hall RC, Chapman MJ. Psychiatric complications of anabolic steroid abuse. Psychosomatics 2005;46:285–90.

[55] Trenton AJ, Currier GW. Behavioural manifestations of anabolic steroid use. CNS Drugs 2005;19:571–95.

[56] McDuff DR, Baron D. Substance use in athletics: a sports psychiatry perspective. Clin Sports Med 2005;24:885–97.

[57] Clark AS, Henderson LP. Behavioral and physiological responses to anabolic-androgenic steroids. Neurosci Biobehav Rev 2003;27:413–36.

[58] Cafri G, Thompson K, Riciardelli L, et al. Pursuit of the muscular ideal: physical and psychological consequences and putative risk factors. Clin Psychol Rev 2005;25:215–39.

[59] Brower KJ, Blow FC, Eliopulos GA, et al. Anabolic androgenic steroids and suicide. Am J Psychiatry 1989;146:1075.

[60] Thiblin I, Runeson B, Rajs J. Anabolic androgenic steroids and suicide. Ann Clin Psychiatry 1999;11:223–31.

[61] Pope HG Jr, Katz DL. Homicide and near-homicide by anabolic steroid users. J Clin Psychiatry 1990;51:28–31.

[62] Fudala PJ, Weinrieb RM, Calarco JS, et al. An evaluation of anabolic-androgenic steroid abusers over a period of 1 year: seven case studies. Ann Clin Psychiatry 2003;15: 121–30.

[63] Conacher GN, Workman DG. Violent crime possibly associated with anabolic steroid use. Am J Psychiatry 1989;146:679.

[64] Pope HG Jr, Katz DL. Psychiatric and medical effects of anabolic-androgenic steroid use. A controlled study of 160 athletes. Arch Gen Psychiatry 1994;51:375–82.

[65] Pope HG Jr, Katz DL. Affective and psychotic symptoms associated with anabolic steroid use. Am J Psychiatry 1988;145:487–90.

[66] Perry PJ, Kutscher EC, Lund BC, et al. Measures of aggression and mood changes in male weightlifters with and without androgenic anabolic steroid use. J Forensic Sci 2003;48: 646–51.

[67] Su TP, Pagliaro M, Schmidt PJ, et al. Neuropsychiatric effects of anabolic steroids in male normal volunteers. JAMA 1993;269:2760–4.

[68] Daly RC, Su TP, Schmidt PJ, et al. Cerebrospinal fluid and behavioral changes after methyltestosterone administration: preliminary findings. Arch Gen Psychiatry 2001;58:172–7.

[69] Pope HG Jr, Kouri EM, Hudson JI. Effects of supraphysiologic doses of testosterone on mood and aggression in normal men: a randomized controlled trial. Arch Gen Psychiatry 2000;57:133–40 [discussion 155–6].

[70] Yates WR, Perry PJ, MacIndoe J, et al. Psychosexual effects of three doses of testosterone cycling in normal men. Biol Psychiatry 1999;45:254–60.

[71] Tricker R, Casaburi R, Storer TW, et al. The effects of supraphysiological doses of testosterone on angry behavior in healthy eugonadal men–a clinical research center study. J Clin Endocrinol Metab 1996;81:3754–8.

[72] Kadi F. Adaptation of human skeletal muscle to training and anabolic steroids. Acta Physiol Scand Suppl 2000;646:1–52.

[73] Kadi F, Bonnerud P, Eriksson A, et al. The expression of androgen receptors in human neck and limb muscles: effects of training and self-administration of androgenic-anabolic steroids. Histochem Cell Biol 2000;113(1):25–9.
[74] Vanderschueren D, Vandenput L, Booonen S, et al. Androgens and bone. Endocr Rev 2004; 25(3):389–425.
[75] Cope MR, Ali A, Bayliss NC. Biceps rupture in body builders: three case reports of rupture of the long head of the biceps at the tendon-labrum junction. J Shoulder Elbow Surg 2004; 13(5):580–2.
[76] Laseter JT, Russell JA. Anabolic steroid-induced tendon pathology: a review of the literature. Med Sci Sports Exerc 1991;23(1):1–3.
[77] Stannard JP, Bucknell AL. Rupture of the triceps tendon associated with steroid injections. Am J Sports Med 1993;21:482–5.
[78] Micheli LJ. Overuse injuries in children's sports: the growth factor. Orthop Clin North Am 1983;14:337–60.
[79] Hergenroeder AC. Prevention of sports injuries. Pediatrics 1998;101(6):1057–63.
[80] Webb DR. Strength training in children and adolescents. Pediatr Clin North Am 1990;37(5): 1187–210.
[81] Braseth NR, Allison EJ Jr, Gough JE. Exertional rhabdomyolysis in a body builder abusing anabolic androgenic steroids. Eur J Emerg Med 2001;8(2):155–7.
[82] Daniels JM, van Westerloo DJ, de Hon OM, et al. [Rhabdomyolysis in a bodybuilder using steroids]. Ned Tijdschr Geneeskd 2006;150(19):1077–80 [in Dutch].
[83] Pertusi R, Dickerman RD, McConathy WJ. Evaluation of aminotransferase elevations in a bodybuilder using anabolic steroids: hepatitis or rhabdomyolysis? J Am Osteopath Assoc 2001;101(7):391–4.
[84] Siddique H, Smith JC, Corrall RJM. Reversal of polycythaemia induced by intramuscular androgen replacement using transdermal testosterone therapy [letter]. Clin Endocrinol 2004;60:142–9.
[85] Tangredi JF, Buxton ILO. Hypertension as a complication of topical testosterone therapy. Ann Pharmacother 2001;35:1205–7.
[86] Palacios A, Campfield LA, McClure RD, et al. Effect of testosterone enanthate on hematopoiesis in normal men. Fertil Steril 1983;40:100–4.
[87] Ferenchick G. Are androgenic steroids thrombogenic? N Engl J Med 1990;322:476.
[88] Product Information. Depo-Testosterone. Kalamazoo (MI): Pharmacia & Upjohn Co.; 2002. Available at: www.pfizer.com/pfizer/download/uspi_depo_testosterone.pdf. Accessed May 27, 2007.
[89] Product Information. Delatestryl. Iselin (NJ): BTG Pharmaceuticals; 1995.
[90] Klasco RK, editor. Poisindex® System. Thomson Micromedex, Greenwood Village, CO. v131, edition expires 3/2007.
[91] American College of Sports Medicine. Position stand: the use of anabolic-androgenic steroids in sports. Med Sci Sports Exerc 1987;19:534–9.
[92] Rich JD, Dickinson BP, Flanigan TP, et al. Abscess related to anabolic-androgenic steroid injection. Med Sci Sports Exerc 1999;31(2):207–9.

Erythropoietin and Other Blood-Boosting Methods

Thomas L. Pommering, DO[a,b,c,*]

[a]*Departments of Pediatrics and Family Medicine, The Ohio State University College of Medicine, Columbus, OH, USA*
[b]*Sports Medicine Program, Columbus Children's Hospital, Columbus, OH, USA*
[c]*Tour de Grandview Professional Cycling Race, Columbus, OH, USA*

Why do athletes use performance-enhancing substances (PESs)? It is not a new phenomenon. PESs have been a part of sports competition since as early as 776 BC when Olympians used substances, such as mushrooms, dried figs, and strychnine, to gain an advantage [1]. Later, heroin, cocaine, and morphine were added and probably did more harm than enhancement [2,3]. Yet, modern athletes are still willing to risk their health, reputation, and even their team or country's honor to gain an athletic advantage.

Nothing illustrates this better than an often-referenced survey published in 1997 in which Olympic hopefuls were asked two simple questions: The first, "If you were offered a banned performance-enhancing substance that guaranteed that you would win an Olympic medal and you would not be caught, would you take it?". Remarkably, 98% of the 198 athletes surveyed reported "yes." But even more remarkable was the answer to the second question, "Would you take a banned performance-enhancing drug that guaranteed you would win an Olympic medal and you will not be caught, you win every competition for the next 5 years, but then will die from adverse effects of the substance?" More than 50% of the athletes still reported "yes" [1,4–6].

The word "doping" was used in the 1860s to describe a drug used for horse racing that consisted of opium and narcotics [7]. With human athletes, "blood doping" originally referred to a process whereby athletes increased their oxygen-carrying capacity by receiving blood transfusions from previously donated blood to increase their hematocrits a few days before competition [5]. The first report of blood doping in a controlled experiment was reported in

---

* Children's Sports Medicine Center, 584 County Line Road West, Westerville, OH 43082.

E-mail address: pommert@pediatrics.ohio-state.edu

1947 [8,9]. Today, "blood doping" is used more synonymously with cheating of any kind, including any of the various blood-boosting methods or classes of ergogenic aids that are available to athletes. Advances in genetic medicine have allowed athletes to raise their level of sophistication significantly by using PESs that are virtually undetectable. The most ubiquitous illegal method of increasing oxygen-carrying capacity in athletes is by the use of recombinant human erythropoietin (rHuEPO). If athletes are caught using rHuEPO, sanctions can range from 2-year suspensions to lifetime bans from competition.

The role of oxygen transport in athletic performance

The body's oxygen transport system brings oxygen to working muscle through a cooperative effort of the circulatory and respiratory systems. There are two ways to improve oxygen transport. The first is to stimulate the natural oxygen carrier, hemoglobin (Hb). The second way is to use other types of oxygen carriers to fill the role of Hb [10]. Athletic endurance is determined by an athlete's maximum oxygen uptake (Vo_2max); by the 1930s, it was clear that champion endurance athletes had extremely high measurements of Vo_2max [11,12]. By the 1970s, it also was evident to the scientific world that maneuvers that increased total body Hb also increased Vo_2max [12]. The athletic world had been exploiting this fact for at least a decade through the practice of blood doping [5,13]. Hence, the modern era of scientifically based performance enhancement for athletes was born.

Physiology of erythropoietin

Structure and function

Erythropoietin (EPO) is a naturally occurring glycoprotein hormone that regulates red blood cell (RBC) production. The peritubular fibroblast cells of the renal cortex produce 90% of the body's EPO, whereas mainly the liver, but also the brain, uterus, and lung account for the remaining 10% [9,14,15]. Within the bone marrow, EPO binds various receptor sites, of which colony-forming unit erythroid cells seem to be most sensitive [16,17]. Subsequently, progenitor cells proliferate into normoblasts and eventually, reticulocytes. Regulation of EPO is controlled by a gene on chromosome 7 (band7q21). The transcription of this gene is controlled by hypoxic inducible factor, which responds to tissue hypoxia [15,18]. Strenuous exercise alone does not seem to affect EPO levels significantly [16]. New circulating erythrocytes are seen within 1 to 2 days after plasma EPO levels increase [14].

Clinical applications

In June 1989, the first rHuEPO product was marketed in the United States. It was isolated and purified from Chinese hamster ovaries and reproduced using DNA recombinant techniques [18]. Until recently, there were two forms of rHuEPO commercially available in the United States: epoetin alfa and epoetin beta. Now, there are at least four erythropoietic isoforms available worldwide that are synthesized by modifying the rHuEPO molecule.

rHuEPO is used to treat anemias related to renal failure, chemotherapy, HIV infection, prematurity, hemoglobinopathies, autoimmune disease, and malignancies, and it is used in patients who undergo surgery who are not candidates for blood transfusion (eg, Jehovah's Witness). It can be administered intravenously (IV) or subcutaneously (SQ). IV dosing results in a shorter half-life and shorter duration of peak plasma levels, which makes SQ administration easier, more effective, and less expensive. The therapeutic range for epoetin alfa is 50 to 300 units/kg given two to three times weekly. Therapeutic increases in hematocrit occur after 2 to 6 weeks, depending on baseline levels and existing iron stores [15,18].

Adverse effects

The most common side effects are headache, fever, nausea, anxiety, and lethargy. Hypertension and hyperkalemia are seen in up to half of patients who are on dialysis [18]. More concerning side effects are associated with hyperviscosity syndromes related to high hematocrits and include myocardial infarction, seizure, stroke and other thromboembolic events, and sudden death [18–21]. When combined with dehydration, athletes are especially at risk for this potentially lethal scenario (see later discussion). Finally, another rare, but serious, side effect is an autoimmune form of pure red cell aplasia that has been linked with SQ administration of rHuEPO [18,22].

Recombinant human erythropoietin

Tainted history

The popularity and effectiveness of rHuEPO in elite endurance athletes is demonstrated by a long list of anecdotes associated with its misuse during international competition. When the average speed of the cyclists racing in the Tour de France began to increase suddenly during the 1990s, rumors of rHuEPO use began to circulate. The gene that produces EPO was cloned in 1985, and rHuEPO was available in Europe by 1987 [23]. Between 1987 and 1991, more than 20 Dutch and Belgian cyclists died at rest—some of them while sleeping—as a result of unexplainable cardiac arrest [13,14,24]. Between 1997 and 2000, 18 more cyclists died from pulmonary embolisms, stroke, and myocardial infraction [5]. Finally, suspicions of rHuEPO use in professional cyclists competing in Europe were confirmed during the 1998 Tour de France; boxes of ampules containing rHuEPO were found in team vehicles and the personal rooms of riders from many of the biggest and most successful teams [14]. It became embarrassingly clear that rHuEPO use in elite professional cyclists was organized, widespread, and sophisticated.

Ergogenic effectiveness of recombinant human erythropoietin

The ability of rHuEPO to enhance endurance is impressive. Athletes can improve their overall performance by as much as 10% to 15% [25]. Although there is a paucity of literature documenting the ergogenic potential of rHuEPO in elite athletes, what has been published using moderately trained subjects shows similarly effective results when comparing rHuEPO with RBC infusion [5]. Specifically, Ekblom and Berglund [26] showed similar increases in Vo$_2$max and time to exhaustion on a treadmill run after several weeks of rHuEPO administration compared with an acute infusion of RBCs. In addition, Audran and colleagues [27] demonstrated a significant increase in Vo$_2$max, ventilatory threshold, and a decrease in maximal heart rate after only 25 days of rHuEPO administration.

Detection of recombinant human erythropoietin

The International Olympic Committee (IOC) added rHuEPO to its list of banned substances in 1990, even though all forms of blood doping had been officially prohibited since 1984 [17,28,29]. The use of rHuEPO also is banned by the US Olympic Committee and the National Collegiate Athletic Association [18]. The challenges associated with detecting rHuEPO lie in the fact that it is almost identical in structure and metabolism to endogenous erythropoietin and it has a rapid half-life (4–9 hours for IV administration and 24 hours for SQ administration), allowing it to clear the body within 2 to 3 days [18,29,30].

Despite justified suspicions of rHuEPO use in cycling and the inability of current methods to detect its use [31], in 1997, the governing body of the International Cycling Union (UCI) enacted hematocrit cutoffs for male (50%) and female (47%) cyclists while more reliable methods of detection could be developed [14,18]. The hematocrit cutoffs were based on existing normative data on elite athletes, taking into consideration the expected effect of dehydration, in an attempt not to exclude athletes with normal variations but to protect athletes from danger [32]. Anyone over that limit would be considered "unfit to race" and could not compete for 2 weeks, although they were not subjected to official sanctions.

To circumvent this, an athlete could inject rHuEPO every 2 to 3 days over 3 to 4 weeks, along with some form of iron supplementation, to get a desired effect and then reduce the dose to match the basal rate of endogenous EPO production to maintain one's hematocrit just below the "legal limit."

During the 2000 Sydney Olympics, the IOC approved the use of a test developed by the Australian Institute of Sport to detect rHuEPO users.

The test relied on mathematical models applied to the measurements of indirect blood markers associated with rHuEPO use, such as soluble transferrin, reticulocyte percentage, and EPO or Hb levels. This test produced an "ON-model" that was designed to identify current or recent users and an "OFF-model" for users weeks after stopping treatment [14,17,33,34,35]. Although this method was quick, inexpensive, and could use existing technology, it had some major drawbacks, one of which was the fact that a required "B" blood sample could not be preserved reliably for confirmatory testing at a later date because of the instability of whole blood, even with freezing. Thus, it was used only as a screen to decide when to apply a new test—the Lasne test, developed earlier that year—that specifically could detect rHuEPO in the urine [36].

Just before the 2000 Sydney Olympics, the National Anti-Doping Laboratory in France developed a direct test for rHuEPO that is based on the fact that the exogenous isoforms of rHuEPO are slightly more acidic than endogenous EPO [36]. Using two techniques—isoelectric focusing and immunoblotting—it was possible to distinguish between natural EPO and the four current isoforms of synthetic EPO plus a newer analog, darbopoietin. Disadvantages of the test are that it is labor intensive, taking 3 days to obtain a final result [35], and expensive, at least $130 per test [31]. Also, because of the short half-life of rHuEPO, the urine sample has to be collected within 2 to 3 days of rHuEPO use to be accurate [18,31]. More recently, researchers reported on a false positive detection in a postexercise, protein-rich urine sample [37]. To the author's current knowledge, this is still the test of choice for detecting rHuEPO use in elite athletes.

Other blood-boosting methods

High-altitude training and altitude tents

Oxygen binding to Hb is determined by the partial pressure of oxygen in the plasma (pO2). Additionally, in environments of low pO2, Hb modifies itself to bind oxygen more efficiently [9]. Using this concept, altitude is used as a natural stimulus for erythropoiesis. It requires 3 to 4 weeks before a response is seen [10] and is "legal." Despite a paucity of randomized, controlled studies, some form of this technique ("sleep high and train low" or vice versa) is practiced often by elite endurance athletes. For those athletes who are geographically challenged, hypobaric chambers or tents that simulate altitudes of 9000 to 13,000 feet can be purchased for about $5000 to $10,000.

Blood doping

During the 1967 Olympics in Mexico, an elite cyclist broke the outdoor 1-hour cycling record. He was reported to have been accompanied by an entourage of two cardiologists and eight men aged 18 to 20 years, chosen several months before the games because of their blood type compatibility

[9]. Autologous or heterologous blood transfusions were used most prevalently by athletes during the 1970s and 1980s, until the risk for blood-borne infections became more apparent. The IOC banned this practice in 1976 [10]. With the Lasne test now available, this practice has resurfaced as an option for some athletes. Currently, only heterologous blood transfusions are detectable.

Novel erythropoiesis-stimulating protein (darbepoietin)

Novel erythropoiesis-stimulating protein was developed by increasing the carbohydrate content of EPO, giving it a longer half-life and enhanced biologic activity, and, thus, allowing less frequent injections [9,10]. The result is an EPO analog named darbepoietin. Three athletes were excluded from the Olympic Games at Salt Lake City for darbepoietin use [10].

Artificial oxygen carriers

Artificial oxygen carriers or blood substitutes were designed to serve as a temporary replacement for transfused RBCs. Their potential clinical applications include RBC replacement during surgery and emergency resuscitation and as a therapeutic adjunct treatment for chemotherapy [38]. Although banned in international competition, these agents are not tested for routinely, except during exceptional circumstances [10]. Elite cyclists are notorious for their abuse. They are classified into two general categories: hemoglobin oxygen carriers (HBOCs) and perfluorocarbon emulsions (PFCs).

Hemoglobin oxygen carriers

Several HBOCs are available for human and veterinary use. There is little published data on the human ergogenic potential of HBOCs [38]. One recent study did not find a significantly positive effect on endurance performance or Vo_2max with one particular form of HBOC, but it did describe hypertension as a significant side effect [39]. Other known adverse affects include gastrointestinal hypertonicity and potentially fatal renal toxicity [38].

Perfluorocarbon emulsions

Chemically related to the commercial product, Teflon, this chemically inert synthetic liquid can dissolve oxygen more than 100 times per equal volume of plasma [38]. This was demonstrated spectacularly in 1966 when a rat was able to survive for hours while totally immersed in an oxygen-saturated PFC solution [38,40]. Without concomitant oxygen supplementation, PFCs likely would not benefit endurance athletes [10]. Side effects include flu-like symptoms, thrombocytopenia, allergic reactions—and more seriously—hepatosplenomegaly, organ failure, and immune compromise (because PFCs are inert and can only be removed by the reticuloendothelial system) [38].

Gene doping

Gene doping was added to the prohibited list by the World Anti-Doping Agency in 2005 and was defined as the "non-therapeutic use of cells, genes, genetic elements, or modulation of gene expression, having the capacity to enhance human performance" [41,42]. This can be accomplished with the use of biologic vectors (viruses), chemical sources (liposomes), or physical methods (direct injection of gene) [41]. As with all forms of gene doping, the potential problem with EPO gene therapy is with gene overexpression leading to excessive erythropoiesis and its deadly consequences. Gene doping is expected to be seen by the 2008 Beijing Olympic Games [29,41,43]. There are no effective ways to identify or prevent gene doping.

The reality

Current testing for rHuEPO or other advanced blood-boosting techniques is inadequate and easy for athletes to "beat." The "dopers" continue to stay a few steps ahead of the "testers." Drug testing is extremely expensive, and its methods are subject to the rigors of scientific validation to protect the athletes who are competing fairly. Funding challenges for new tests and barriers to testing still exist [26,44]. Perhaps a more reasonable approach is for elite athletes to have a type of "hematologic passport" [34], coupled with longitudinal laboratory monitoring, to document where athletes' normal or "clean" baseline hematologic parameters should be [17,45]. As this article was being written, professional cycling teams are adopting this policy in a first sincere attempt by a team owner in professional cycling to clean up the sport. Although there remains the tremendous financial incentives attached to success in sports competition, there will always dangle the "doping carrot."

Final thoughts

For now, the use of rHuEPO in young athletes is not believed to be nearly as prevalent as with their adult counterparts; however, it is known that young users typically minimize the known health risks associated with using ergogenic aids, which puts them at particular risk for future use and subsequent harm [46]. Early recognition by physicians, parents, and coaches followed by honest education and "thoughtful discouragement" has been recommended as a strategy to dissuade adolescents away from ergogenic aids [46–48].

Some investigators have advocated a position that by allowing and monitoring PESs, the athlete's health and safety would be improved [3]. This philosophy should be denounced; it would give young athletes and their supporters a new, unparalleled, and seemingly legitimate incentive to risk their health in their quest for the opportunity of future sporting success. As physicians, parents, and coaches, how would we then counsel our young athletes?

Summary

The use of rHuEPO to illegally enhance performance and its health risks are well documented. Testing methods exist, but they can easily be outwitted. Today's athletes also can choose from other blood-boosting methods and often use these concomitantly with rHuEPO. Most notable is the emerging genetic technology, which may, as soon as the 2008 Olympic Games, antiquate all other "doping" methods as athletes continue to place themselves at the ultimate risk in search of success and glory.

References

[1] Calfee R, Fadale P. Popular ergogenic drugs and supplements in young athletes. Pediatrics 2006;117(3):577–89.

[2] Noakes TD. Tainted glory-doping and athletic performance. N Engl J Med 2004;351(9): 847–9.

[3] Savulescu J, Foddy B, Clayton M. Why we should allow performance enhancing drugs in sport. Br J Sports Med 2004;38:66–70.

[4] Bamberger M, Yeager D. Over the edge: special report. Sports Illustrated 1997;18:268–80.

[5] Tokish JM, Kocher MS, Hawkins RJ. Ergogenic aids: a review of basic science, performance, side effects, and status in sports. Am J Sports Med 2004;32(6):1543–53.

[6] Congeni J, Miller S. Supplements and drugs used to enhance athletic performance. Pediatr Clin North Am 2002;49:435–61.

[7] Pabinger C, Gruber G. World anti-doping regulations for 2005: essential changes for athletes and physicians. Arch Orthop Trauma Surg 2006;126:286–8.

[8] Pace N. The increase in hypoxia tolerance of normal men accompanying the polycythemia induced by transfusion of erythrocytes. Am J Physiol 1947;148:152–63.

[9] Fisher JW. Erythropoietin: physiology and pharmacology update. Exp Biol Med (Maywood) 2003;228:1–14.

[10] Gaudard A, Varlet-Marie E, Bressole F, et al. Drugs for increasing oxygen transport and their potential use in doping. A review. Sports Med 2003;33(3):187–212.

[11] Robinson S, Edwards HT, Dill DB. New records in human power. Science 1937;85:409–10.

[12] Joyner MJ. VO$_2$max, blood doping, and erythropoietin. Br J Sports Med 2003;37:190–1.

[13] Ciocca M. Medication and supplement use by athletes. Clin Sports Med 2005;24:719–38.

[14] Bento RM, Damasceno LM, Neto FR. Recombinant human erythropoietin in sports: a review. Rev Bras Med Esporte 2003;9(3):181–90.

[15] Marsden JT. Erythropoietin-measurement and clinical applications. Ann Clin Biochem 2006;43:97–104.

[16] Jelkmann W. Erythropoietin. J Endocrinol Invest 2003;26:832–7.

[17] Robinson N, Giraud S, Baume N, et al. Erythropoietin and blood doping. Br J Sports Med 2006;40(Suppl I):I30–4.

[18] Scott J, Phillips GC. Erythropoietin in sports: a new look at an old problem. Curr Sports Med Rep 2005;4(4):224–6.

[19] Greydanus DE, Patel DR. Sports doping in the adolescent athlete. The hope, hype and hyperbole. Pediatr Clin North Am 2002;49:829–55.

[20] Patel DR, Greydanus DE, Luckstead EF. The college athlete. Pediatr Clin North Am 2005; 52:25–60.

[21] Koch JJ. Performance-enhancing substances and their use among adolescent athletes. Pediatr Rev 2002;23(9):310–7.

[22] Cazzola M. Erythropoietin therapy: need for rationality and active surveillance. Haematologica 2003;88(6):601–4.

[23] Ellender L, Linder MM. Sports pharmacology and ergogenic aids. Prim Care Clin Office Pract 2005;32:277–92.
[24] Vogel G. A race to the starting line. Science 2004;305(5684):632–5.
[25] Birchard K. Past, present, and future of drug abuse at the Olympics. Lancet 2000;356:1008.
[26] Ekblom B, Berglund B. Effect of erythropoietin on maximal aerobic power. Scand J Med Sci Sports 1991;1:88–93.
[27] Audran M, Gareau R, Matecki S, et al. Effects of erythropoietin administration in training athletes and possible indirect detection in doping control. Med Sci Sports Exerc 1999;31(5):639–45.
[28] Diamanti-Kandarakis E, Konstantinopoulos PA, Papailiou J, et al. Erythropoietin abuse and erythropoietin gene doping. Sports Med 2005;35(10):831–40.
[29] Lippi G, Guidi G. Laboratory screening for erythropoietin abuse in sport: an emerging challenge. Clin Chem Lab Med 2000;38(1):13–9.
[30] Abbott A. What price the Olympian idea? Nature 2000;407:124–7.
[31] Birkland KI, Donike M, Ljungqvist A, et al. Blood sampling in doping control: first experiences from regular testing in athletics. Int J Sports Med 1997;18(1):7–12.
[32] Saris WHM, Senden JMG, Brouns F. What is the normal red-blood cell mass for professional cyclists? Lancet 1998;352:1758.
[33] Cazzola M. A strategy to deter blood doping in sport. Haematologica 2002;87(3):225–34.
[34] Pascual JA, Belalcazar V, de Bolos C, et al. Recombinant erythropoietin and analogues: a challenge for doping control. Ther Drug Monit 2004;26(2):175–9.
[35] Gore CJ, Parisotto R, Ashenden MJ, et al. Second-generation blood tests to detect erythropoietin abuse by athletes. Haemotologica 2003;88:333–44.
[36] Lasne F, Ceaurriz J. Recombinant erythropoietin in urine. Nature 2000;405:635.
[37] Beullens M, Delanghe JR, bollen M. False-positive detection of recombinant human erythropoietin in urine following strenuous physical exercise. Blood 2006;107(12):4711–3.
[38] Schumacher YO, Ashenden M. Doping with artificial oxygen carriers: an update. Sports Med 2004;34(3):141–50.
[39] Ashenden MJ, Schumacher YO, Sharpe K, et al. Effects of hemopure™ on maximal oxygen uptake and endurance performance in healthy humans. Int J Sports Med 2007;28(5):381–5.
[40] Clark LC, Gollan R. Survival of animals breathing organic liquids equilibrated with oxygen at atmospheric pressure. Science 1966;152:1755–6.
[41] Azzazy H, Mansour M, Christenson RH. Doping in the recombinant era: strategies and counterstrategies. Clin Biochem 2005;38:959–65.
[42] World Anti-Doping Agency. Available at: http://www.wada-ama.org. Accessed February 1, 2007.
[43] Adam D. Gene therapy may be up to speed for cheats at 2008 Olympics. Nature 2001;414:569–70.
[44] Zorpette G. All doped up-and going for the gold. Sci Am 2000;282(5):20–2.
[45] Sharpe K. A third generation approach to detect erythropoietin abuse in athletes. Haematologica 2006;91(3):356–63.
[46] Laure P, Lecerf T, Friser A, et al. Drugs, recreational drug use and attitudes towards doping in high school students. Int J Sports Med 2004;25:133–8.
[47] Laos C, Metzl JD. Performance-enhancing drug use in young athletes. Adolesc Med 2006;17:719–31.
[48] Hampton T. Researchers address use of performance-enhancing drugs in elite athletes. JAMA 2006;295(6):607–8.

ELSEVIER
SAUNDERS

PEDIATRIC CLINICS

OF NORTH AMERICA

Pediatr Clin N Am 54 (2007) 701–711

The World Anti-Doping Program and the Primary Care Physician

Richard L. Hilderbrand, PhD

United States Anti-Doping Agency, 1330 Quail Lake Loop,
Suite 260, Colorado Springs, CO 80906, USA

Over the past 4 decades, the role of the physician in the treatment of athletes has changed significantly. The traditional role of the physician in sport was the immediate protection of the health of the athlete, including treatment of injuries and illness. Unfortunately, some physicians have crossed the line from legitimately restoring health to the improper use of medications to enhance performance. This may happen because the line is not always clear, especially in the presence of the growth of preventive and wellness medicine, or it may be the result of a rogue physician working with an athlete to achieve improper objectives. In any case, the role of physicians in aiding athletes who want to dope has expanded [1,2]. With the pharmaceutical and technological developments of the recent past, the athletes who are doping (Box 1) have become dependent on physicians and other medical professionals to achieve their maximum results. This is a matter of grave concern, and the US Anti-Doping Agency (USADA) is working with medical professionals and others to establish ethical standards on the treatment of athletes.

Conversely, the role of the physician in anti-doping efforts has increased remarkably, as well. The greatest change has taken place in the last few years, with primary care physicians and specialists having a formalized role in submitting documentation to support an athlete's request to use medications that may be prohibited in sport [3]. The International Standard for Therapeutic Use Exemptions (TUEs) [4] is a part of the World Anti-Doping Code (the Code) [5] and allows an athlete who has a legitimate medical need for the use of an otherwise prohibited substance to submit a request to use that particular medication. There are two types of TUEs that are used for two different purposes: the Abbreviated TUE and the Standard TUE. If filled out properly and completely, the Abbreviated TUE, which is a notification only, is effective upon receipt at the responsible anti-doping

E-mail address: rhilderbrand@usantidoping.org

doi:10.1016/j.pcl.2007.04.005   *pediatric.theclinics.com*

Box 1. Definition of doping as defined in the Code

The presence of a prohibited substance, or its metabolites or
markers, in an athlete's bodily specimen (the athlete is
responsible for any prohibited substance that is in his/her
system, irrespective of how the substance got into the body).

Use or attempted use of a prohibited substance or a prohibited
method. The use does not have to be successful to be a doping
violation.

Refusing, or failing without compelling justification, to submit to
sample collection after appropriate notification.

Not being available for testing as a result of failure to provide
location information or by missing a test.

Tampering, or attempting to tamper, with any part of doping
control.

Possession of prohibited substances. This includes possession
by athletes or support personnel.

Trafficking in any prohibited substance or prohibited method.

Administration, or attempted administration, or assisting,
encouraging, aiding, abetting, covering up, or any other
complicity in an antidoping rule violation.

---

organization. The Abbreviated TUE applies only to corticosteroids administered by inhalation or local injection and certain β-2 agonists that are permitted by inhalation for respiratory conditions. The Abbreviated TUE relies
on the signature of the physician and only rarely requires medical record
documentation. The Standard TUE, which applies to all other prohibited
substances and methods, must be supported by complete medical documentation. The Standard TUE must be submitted and approved before the use
of the prohibited medication or method in sport. These two exemption request forms are covered in detail in the next section. Because the procedures
and documentation that are required by sport authorities are complex, this
article is intended to provide explanatory information and specific assistance
to pediatricians and primary care providers, in general, on how to comply
with the rules that apply under the Code. Now, more than in the past, physicians must be involved in the process of doping control.

Anti-Doping organizations

The World Anti-Doping Agency (WADA) was established by the International Olympic Committee (IOC) in November of 1999 as a foundation
with the support and participation of intergovernmental organizations,
governments, public authorities, and other public and private bodies [6].
WADA's mission is to work with the IOC, national anti-doping

organizations (NADO), sports federations, and athletes with the common objective of controlling doping in sport.

USADA is the United States-based NADO; it began operations on October 1, 2000 with full authority for testing, education, research, and results management for US Olympic, Pan American, and Paralympic athletes [7]. WADA and USADA are independent of the bodies responsible as advocates for the advancement of sport.

The World Anti-Doping Program

The objective of the World Anti-Doping Program (the Program) [8] is to preserve what is intrinsically valuable about sport or "the spirit of sport." The spirit of sport is characterized by development of ethics, fair play, honesty, a healthy lifestyle, character, and an ability to participate on a team. An inherent part of character is for the athlete to develop respect for rules, laws, self, and other participants.

The Program consists of the Code, International Standards, and Models of Best Practice. All organizations that are signatories to the Code must follow the Code and the International Standards; the procedures in the Models of Best Practice are recommended. Of particular interest here are the Prohibited List International Standard (2007) [9] and TUEs [4]. The other International Standards are for Laboratories [10] and for Testing [11] of athletes.

The International Standards

Prohibited list

The Prohibited List (the List) is a list of categories of substances and methods that are controlled by WADA. The prohibition may be at all times or only in competition. The List is not exhaustive in that several categories of substances are "open" and include "other substances with a similar chemical structure or similar biological effect(s)." The placement of a substance or method on the List is not subject to appeal by the athlete in the case of a doping violation. The List is compiled by a committee convened by WADA and is updated annually, or more frequently, as needed. Sport-specific prohibitions occur as well (Box 2).

Therapeutic Use Exemptions

The Code permits an athlete to apply for a TUE to use an otherwise prohibited substance or method for a documented therapeutic purpose. The International Standard includes the criteria for allowing the exemption, the application process, and a procedure for appeals to decisions. The ultimate objective is to harmonize this exemption process across the world.

Box 2. Prohibited list of pharmaceuticals, substances, and methods

Substances and methods prohibited at all times (in and out of competition)
Prohibited substances
  Anabolic agents
  Hormones and related substances
  β-2 Agonists
  Agents with antiestrogenic activity
  Diuretics and other masking agents
Prohibited methods
  Enhancement of oxygen transfer
  Chemical and physical manipulation
  Gene doping

Substances prohibited in competition (must be cleared from the body at the competition)
Stimulants
Narcotics
Cannabinoids
Glucocorticosteroids

Substances prohibited in particular sports
Alcohol
β-Blockers

Testing

The testing standard is to plan for effective testing (sample collections) and to maintain the integrity and identity of the samples from the notification of the athlete to receipt of the sample at the laboratory. The topics included are test distribution planning, notification of athletes, processes for collection, security, and transport of samples.

Laboratories

This standard is intended to harmonize the laboratories across the world that are accredited by WADA. The standard, including all annexes and technical documents, is intended to ensure that quality results are produced by all accredited laboratories and that evidentiary data are appropriate for the intended use. The standard also describes the application and accreditation process for the laboratories and the process for accreditation of satellite laboratories created for a specific purpose.

Models of best practice

Models of best practice are based on the Code and are developed to provide the best available information on various areas of anti-doping program operation. These best practices are recommended but not mandatory.

History of medical exemptions to use prohibited medications

With the addition of commonly used pharmaceuticals to the list of prohibited substances that was established by the IOC came the need for elite athletes to use those medications for legitimate medical purposes. In the late 1980s, Sweden and Australia began a process to approve such use of prohibited medications for national athletes. At the 1988 Olympic Games, the IOC Medical Commission allowed the use of oral glucocorticosteroids by a hockey player in Calgary and the use of furosemide by a female heavyweight rower in Seoul. In October of 1991, the IOC established a committee consisting of Drs. Ken Fitch (Chair), Don Catlin, and Arne Ljungvist to prepare criteria by which medical exemptions would be granted. Subsequently, the committee became the Medication Advisory Committee (MAC) of the IOC and continued to make decisions for various Olympic Games and sports until 2002. Following a series of meetings of the MAC with the IOC legal staff, the concept of TUEs was included in the Olympic Movement Anti-Doping Code in 2000. Also in 2000, the concept of TUEs was included in the Olympic Games Doping Control Guide for the Sydney Olympic Games. After the Games, the Australian TUE Committee prepared a protocol for TUEs. This was the basis for the TUE process that was adopted at the World Conference on Doping in Sport in Copenhagen, Denmark on March 5, 2003 and promulgated as an International Standard in 2004 [12].

Therapeutic Use Exemptions

The authority to review and accept an Abbreviated or Standard TUE [5] is established by the Code [6]. An International Federation (IF) is established for each sport (eg, the International Ski Federation is the IF for skiing) and writes and updates the rules of competition for elite national, international, and Olympic sport competitions. The Code gives the IFs responsibility for receiving and approving TUEs for international-level athletes or those athletes who compete at international events. USADA is given responsibility for receiving and approving TUEs for American national-level athletes. The IFs may retain the review of the TUE requests made by international-level athletes or they may agree with organizations (eg, USADA) to have the decisions made at the national level. Unless there is an agreement in place that an IF will recognize the decision of a national-level anti-doping body (such as USADA), any national-level athletes who move to international competition must ensure that the TUE request to the appropriate IF for their sport is completed in a timely manner and before they might be subject to doping control.

There are several salient points related to the TUE process that medical care providers need to be aware of. First, USADA does not provide advice on medical matters or treatments. Treatment for routine or emergency medical conditions is between the athlete and his/her physician. The athlete is responsible for managing his/her own care and for using medications in a manner consistent with the Code [5]. The anti-doping rules do not deny or recommend the use of medications, they only control how the medications may be used in sport. USADA provides information on the status of medications solely for athletes' information, in accordance with the Code. Second, anti-doping rules, like competition rules, are rules governing conditions under which sport is played and must be complied with in the same manner as rules on the field of play, equipment, time, and so forth. Please remember that prohibited substances (eg, methylphenidate, oral methylprednisolone, insulin, or oxandrolone) used to treat a legitimate medical condition (without a TUE) are prohibited even if prescribed properly by a medical professional.

Abbreviated Therapeutic Use Exemptions

The Abbreviated TUE only applies to in-competition and out-of-competition use of four β-2 agonists (formoterol, salbutamol [also known as albuterol or levalbuterol], salmeterol, and terbutaline) by inhalation and the in-competition use of glucocorticosteroids by inhalation and local or intra-articular injection. An Abbreviated TUE for use of any of the four listed β-2 agonists must be received prior to the athlete being tested in- or out-of-competition (Box 3).

Standard Therapeutic Use Exemptions

A Standard TUE may be requested for the use of an otherwise prohibited substance and for which an Abbreviated TUE is not allowed [4]. International-level athletes may send the completed application to USADA for forwarding to the appropriate IF. National-level athletes must submit the Standard TUE to USADA. In cases in which IF approval is needed, USADA forwards the request. USADA has established the required processes for reviewing the Standard TUEs, including a Therapeutic Use Exemption Committee (TUEC) for review and an appeal process for national-level athletes.

The Standard TUE application must include a comprehensive medical history and the results of all examinations, laboratory investigations, and imaging studies relevant to the diagnosis that is the basis for the request. Any additional relevant investigations, examinations, or imaging studies requested by the TUEC will be at the expense of the athlete

---

Box 3. Summary of requirements for an acceptable Abbreviated Therapeutic Use Exemption

The correct Abbreviated TUE form must be completed fully. For example, certain IFs require the use of their own form.

All information written on the form must be legible (to allow faxing and understanding by the international medical community). Typed or block letters are preferred.

The generic name, rather than the brand name (for example, salbutamol rather than Ventolin), is needed. These forms will be faxed to IFs and WADA, and brand names differ from country to country.

All signatures (parent/guardian as applicable) and address information for the athlete and physician must be included.

All medical information on the β-2 agonists or glucocorticosteroids including, but not limited to, diagnosis, medical examinations performed (including dates), dose, route of administration, frequency of use, and duration of treatment with the prohibited substances must be included.

Failure to follow these instructions will delay the processing of the request.

---

making the request. The application must be legible, signed by an appropriately qualified physician, and describe the necessity of the otherwise prohibited substance or prohibited method. In particular, the need for the prohibited substance must be justified, and the reasons why alternative permitted medications cannot, or could not, be used also must be cited. The dose, frequency, route, and duration of administration of the otherwise prohibited substance or prohibited method must be specified. If a TUE has been granted to an athlete by USADA, the athlete and WADA are promptly provided with a notification of approval and information pertaining to the duration and any conditions associated with the TUE. Standard TUEs may be considered for renewal by submission of a new form with medical information to update the record from the last submission. Some IFs may require a complete resubmission for a renewal.

Emergency Therapeutic Use Exemptions

In certain emergency situations in which a prohibited substance or method is required to protect the health of the athlete and there is insufficient time to file the appropriate Standard or Abbreviated TUE, an Emergency TUE may be filed. The Emergency TUE, in all cases, requires the

Standard TUE form with medical documentation supporting the emergency request. An example of an emergency situation is an oral glucocorticosteroid to treat anaphylactic shock. The decision on the Emergency TUE is, of necessity, made after the fact.

Therapeutic Use Exemption Committee review factors

The TUEC considers the request and the medical information submitted. The Committee is not convened to complete a diagnosis or to recommend any treatment plan. The committee is solely tasked with evaluating the application with the existing medical information and to make a determination if the use of the prohibited medications or method falls within the rules of sport. In this process, the Committee first determines that the diagnosis is appropriate and well documented. Several factors are considered; however, the key items are the credentials of the physician completing the request, the types of examination or evaluation used in making the diagnosis, and the acceptability of the documentation. Specialty training of the submitting physician in the area of the diagnosis is a positive factor in the consideration (Boxes 4 and 5).

Appeal of decisions

In the case of the denial of a request for a TUE, international-level United States athletes, those who enter an international competition, or national-level athletes included in the national antidoping organization's Registered Testing Pool may submit a request for a review of the decision. WADA has established a fee that applies to the review of appeals. For information on how to request a review or file an appeal, see Section 7 of the WADA International Standard for Therapeutic Use Exemptions.

In the case of the denial of a request for a TUE by athletes other than those listed above, the athlete may request a review of the decision from

---

Box 4. Criteria used by the Therapeutic Use Exemption Committee

If the athlete would suffer significant impairment without the use of the prohibited medication.

If the medication will produce significant performance. enhancement above what would be obtained with a return to normal health.

If there are reasonable therapeutic alternatives.

If the need is a result of a prior nontherapeutic use of an otherwise prohibited medication or method.

Box 5. Therapeutic Use Exemption Committee requirements for attention deficit disorder/attention-deficit/hyperactivity disorder medications

A thorough clinical history, including the initial reports that led to the diagnosis of attention deficit disorder/attention-deficit/ hyperactivity disorder, discussion of the measures used and their interpretation, age of onset, and family history of related diagnoses.

A description of the deficit in performance, physical or mental, exhibited by the athlete and the description of how the proposed medication will affect performance at the doses used.

The results of any laboratory testing completed during diagnosis.

Any observations and consequences of discontinuance of the medication for a brief period of time.

Evidence that permitted medications have been considered or tried and that the outcome of use of the allowed medications is such that the prohibited medication must be used.

Any clinical, educational, psychologic, or consultative reports with comments on related performance issues, such as anxiety or depression.

A statement provided by the athlete outlining how he/she feels when the medication is being taken and not taken. This statement is helpful to the physicians and should, in fact, be written by the athlete. Statements written by parents over the athlete's signature are not helpful and should not be submitted.

USADA. The review is conducted by an independent physician and is based on the material included in the initial submission of the athlete. There is a fee associated with this request for review. The request must be made within 30 days of the receipt of the decision from the initial TUEC.

Summary

The presence of a prohibited substance in an athlete's urine (or blood, when applicable) or the use of a prohibited method constitutes a doping offense. The presence of a prohibited substance is a violation irrespective of the manner in which the prohibited substance came to be in the athlete's system. It is the personal responsibility of an athlete to ensure that no prohibited substance is allowed to enter his or her body or use, or allow the use of, any prohibited method (in other words, the concept of "strict liability" applies). For the therapeutic use of a prohibited substance or method, the TUE rules must be followed. The TUE must be obtained according to WADA guidelines and before testing or conditions where the substance is prohibited. Ultimately, the most powerful deterrent to doping may be the proactive maintenance of a supportive, open, and trusting professional relationship between athletes and medical personnel. The medical personnel must be perfectly clear that doping practices are seen as ethically unacceptable.

In the past few years, anti-doping programs have been established to have independence from the sport organizations that are expected to be advocates of sport. The World Anti-Doping Program has established International Standards for a Prohibited List (substances and methods) and for Therapeutic Use Exemptions to allow athletes who have essential medical needs to use a prohibited substance or method. In addition, WADA has established International Standards for Testing and for Laboratories and is working to harmonize these programs worldwide. The procedures for requesting TUEs have been developed carefully. These procedures and the criteria for evaluation were presented here in some detail. At this time, the Code is being reviewed and revised and will be formalized at a World Conference in the fall of 2007. Certain minor aspects of the Code and requirements for TUEs may be modified; however, the changes are expected to be minimal. Updated information on the Code, including any revisions to the International Standard for TUEs, may be found on the WADA Web site. In addition, USADA provides information on prohibited substances and the TUE process in a variety of ways. Information on prohibited substances and TUEs is available online at the USADA Drug Reference Online (DRO) [13], by telephone at the Drug Reference Line (DRL) (800-233-0393), and in the *USADA Guide to Prohibited Substances and Prohibited Methods of Doping*, which is available online [14] or in printed format [15]. Given the growing complexity of sports medicine and doping methods, physicians and other support personnel must play an important role in influencing the decisions of athletes that effect long-term health.

Acknowledgments

The author thanks Drs. Larry Bowers and Caroline Hatton for their constructive comments on this article, and Ms. Carla O'Connell and Ms. Camila Zardo for editorial and preparation assistance. Despite the assistance, the author accepts responsibility for any factual errors or misrepresentations that may be included in the writing.

References

[1] Pipe A, Best T. Editorial. Drugs, sport, and medical practice. Clin J Sport Med 2002;12: 201–2.
[2] Hoberman J. Sports physicians and the doping crisis in elite sport. Clin J Sport Med 2002;12: 203–8.
[3] Green G. Doping control for the team physician: a review of drug testing procedures in sport. Am J Sports Med 2006;34:1690–8.

[4] World Anti-Doping Agency. The World Anti-Doping Code. International standard for therapeutic use exemptions. Available at: http://www.wada-ama.org/rtecontent/document/international_standard.pdf. Accessed January 12, 2007.

[5] World Anti-Doping Agency. The World Anti-Doping Code, Version 3. 2003. Available at: http://www.wada-ama.org/rtecontent/document/code_v3.pdf. Accessed January 12, 2007.

[6] Lausanne Declaration on doping in sport. Adopted at the World conference on doping in sport. Lausanne (Switzerland), February 2–4, 1999.

[7] Report of the U.S. Olympic Committee select task force on externalization. Presented at the U.S. Anti-Doping Agency 2001 Annual Report. USADA. Colorado Springs (CO), December 3, 1999.

[8] World Anti-Doping Agency. The World Anti-Doping Agency Mission. Available at: http://www.wada-ama.org/en/dynamic.ch2?pageCategory.id=255. Accessed January 12, 2007.

[9] World Anti-Doping Agency. The World Anti-Doping Code. 2007 Prohibited List, International Standard. Available at: http://www.wada-ama.org/rtecontent/document/2007_List_En.pdf. Accessed January 12, 2007.

[10] World Anti-Doping Agency. International Standard for Laboratories. Available at: http://www.wada-ama.org/rtecontent/document/lab_aug_04.pdf. Accessed January 12, 2007.

[11] World Anti-Doping Agency. The World Anti-Doping Code. International standard for testing. Available at: http://www.wada-ama.org/rtecontent/document/testing_v3_a.pdf. Accessed January 12, 2007.

[12] Fitch K. History of therapeutic use exemptions. Presented at World Anti-Doping Agency/National Anti-Doping Agency Meeting On Therapeutic Use Exemptions. Bonn (Germany), December 13, 2006.

[13] United States Anti-Doping Agency. Drug reference online (DRO). Available at: www.usantidoping.org/dro. Accessed June 12, 2007.

[14] United States Anti-Doping Agency. 2007 Guide to Prohibited Substances and Prohibited Methods of Doping. 7th edition. Available at: http://www.usantidoping.org/files/active/what/usada_guide.pdf. Accessed February 1, 2007.

[15] United States Anti-Doping Agency. Guide to prohibited substances and prohibited methods of doping. 7th edition. Colorado Springs (CO): USADA; 2006.

ELSEVIER
SAUNDERS

Pediatr Clin N Am 54 (2007) 713–733

PEDIATRIC CLINICS

OF NORTH AMERICA

Beyond Sports-Doping Headlines:
The Science of Laboratory Tests
for Performance-Enhancing Drugs

Caroline K. Hatton, PhD

*UCLA Olympic Laboratory, University of California at Los Angeles,
2122 Granville Avenue, Los Angeles, CA 90025, USA*

Young athletes breaking into the elite level can look forward to giving interviews, autographs... and urine samples. This article shows what happens when the latter are tested for prohibited doping agents at the laboratory—how roomfuls of regulations and teams of specialized professionals ensure that the laboratory work is conducted accurately and that the test results are handled properly. Drug testing, along with drug education, research, and results management, is how an antidoping program enforces the rules, protects fair play, and defends the clean athletes' freedom to compete without drugs.

Regulatory framework

The fight against drug abuse in sports has grown and improved since doping control began in the 1960s. Worldwide antidoping efforts are better organized, harmonized, and structured than ever. This is true not only of the rules, prohibited substances and methods, sanctions, and appeals, but also of laboratory accreditation and reporting criteria. A positive test result, or laboratory report that a prohibited drug was found in a sample, is referred to in antidoping jargon as an adverse analytical finding. It is the antidoping organization that determines whether the case is positive.

The World Anti-Doping Agency (WADA, see Box 1 for common acronyms) has the support and participation of World Anti-Doping Code signatories, such as governments and private entities, to work with the International Olympic Committee (IOC), national antidoping organizations (NADOs), sports federations, and athletes to control doping in sport.

E-mail address: ckhatton@aol.com

Box 1. List of acronyms

CIR: carbon isotope ratio (same as carbon IRMS)
DAD: diode array detector
EPO: erythropoietin
ERC: endogenous reference compound
GC: gas chromatography
GC-C-IRMS: gas chromatography-combustion-isotope ratio mass spectrometry
GC-MS: gas chromatography-mass spectrometry
GC-MS-MS: gas chromatography-tandem mass spectrometry
GH: growth hormone
HBOC: hemoglobin-based oxygen carrier
hCG: human chorionic gonadotropin
HES: hydroxyethylstarch
HPLC: high-performance liquid chromatography
IA: immunoassay
IEC: International Electrochemical Commission
IEF: isoelectric focusing
IOC: International Olympic Committee
IRMS: isotope ratio mass spectrometry (when applied to carbon, same as CIR)
ISL: International Standard for Laboratories (WADA)
ISO: the symbolic name of the International Organization for Standardization
LC-MS: liquid chromatography-mass spectrometry
LC-MS-MS: liquid chromatography-tandem mass spectrometry
LH: luteinizing hormone
MRM: multiple reaction monitoring
MS: mass spectrometry
NADO: national antidoping organization
NCAA: National Collegiate Athletic Association
RSR-13: a pharmaceutical hemoglobin modifier
SIM: selected ion monitoring
SOP: standard operating procedure
SRM: selected reaction monitoring
TD: technical document (WADA)
THG: tetrahydrogestrinone
TMS: trimethylsilyl
TUE: Therapeutic Use Exemption
USADA: United States Anti-Doping Agency
WADA: World Anti-Doping Agency

NADOs testing programs, such as that of the US Anti-Doping Agency (USADA), fall under WADA regulations, but those of United States professional sports, the National Collegiate Athletic Association (NCAA), and United States high schools do not.

The WADA 2007 List of Prohibited Substances and Methods [1] includes prohibitions effective at all times or only in competition. Among them are anabolic agents (eg, anabolic steroids), hormones (eg, erythropoietin [EPO]), diuretics, and other masking agents, chemical and physical manipulation, stimulants, and more. The list gives examples in each class and includes "other substances with a similar chemical structure or similar biological effect(s)." Therefore, athletes cannot claim innocence merely because the drug that they used was not listed by name. Only nine of several hundred prohibited drugs have a cut-off [2]; for all the others, any detectable amount constitutes an adverse analytical finding. In the United States, professional sports, the NCAA [3], and high schools have their own prohibited lists, which overlap with those of WADA.

National antidoping agencies, such as USADA, must use WADA-accredited laboratories to test the samples that they collect. A prerequisite to WADA accreditation is ISO accreditation (ie, the laboratory must meet the requirements of ISO/IEC 17025) [4]. These include a quality assurance program, standard operating procedure (SOP) for assays; instrument operation and maintenance; personnel qualifications; restricted access to premises, computers, and electronic records; internal audit trails; and traceability of results to reference standards.

The WADA requirements for laboratories reflect those of ISO and are stated in the International Standard for Laboratories [4] and WADA technical documents. Generally, WADA does not require laboratories to follow prescribed SOPs; instead, laboratories are required to meet performance criteria. For example, laboratories must be able to detect 2 ng/mL of clenbuterol in urine [2]; the sample preparation procedure and analytical techniques are up to each laboratory. WADA requires laboratories to have research activities to optimize tests performance and to keep up with cheaters. WADA accreditation is up for renewal annually.

Sample identity and integrity

The first step in a doping-control urine test is getting an authentic urine sample from the correct person and getting it sealed and documented for shipment to the laboratory. Thus, the first crucial link in the doping-control process is the Doping Control Officer or Sports Drug Testing Collector and his or her staff.

Athletes who enter sports competitions agree to follow the rules—including antidoping rules—from being subjected to doping-control tests to accepting the consequences of a positive test. Athletes selected for a test identify themselves before they urinate in a cup, under direct observation by an official of the same gender. Next, the urine is poured into a pair of bottles, A and B, labeled only with numbers (eg, 963852A and 963852B), and the bottles are sealed. Only the sport organization—not the laboratory—knows which number corresponds to which athlete. Chain of custody paperwork documents who has custody of the samples or where they are locked up, from the moment the bottles are sealed, to their receipt at the laboratory, to the day when they are finally discarded.

Blood is rarely collected in the major United States sports drug-testing programs. At the Olympics, blood is collected, but not as often as urine. For example, at the 2004 Athens Olympics, the laboratory received 2926 urine samples and 691 blood samples [5]. Some federations, such as Union Cycliste Internationale, collect blood before races for health tests (not doping-control tests), and athletes with atypical values deemed medically unsafe (eg, high hematocrit) are not allowed to compete [6].

Testing urine is better than testing blood for most prohibited substances (small molecules, molecular weight less than ~ 800 atomic mass units). Urine collection is noninvasive and yields a large volume of sample, with higher drug concentrations than in blood and with far fewer cells and proteins to complicate extraction.

Is it possible to tamper with the sample containers? Not without leaving evidence of it. Sample integrity is checked and documented upon receipt at the laboratory, by technicians who inspect containers and tamper-evident seals visually, then record whether the chain of custody was intact. The bottles used at the Olympics are sealed with a thick plastic cap over the stopper, and the only way to access the sample is to destroy the cap.

To deter urine substitution, urination is observed. This led to the discovery at the Athens Olympics of a contraption consisting of a bag of clean urine up the rectum and plastic tubing running along the underside of the penis [7].

High school drug-testing programs may test only for street drugs or only for anabolic steroids. In some programs, samples are not split and adverse analytical findings are not reported by individual bottle number, but only in an aggregate fashion, reporting the finding of a drug with no further detail than "in one sample in the batch."

A doping-control laboratory test consists of more than one test

At the laboratory (Fig. 1), all "A" samples (a portion or "aliquot" of each) undergo screening for all of the drugs on the relevant (in- or out-of-competition) list (menu). The goal of screening is to rapidly sort samples into two categories: certainly negative and maybe containing a target compound. A well-designed screen is quick, detects a broad variety of substances, and provides a mere indication, not full proof, that the compound is present. Because drugs tend to be chemically similar within each class (eg, stimulants,

"ALIQUOT" (= transfer some urine)...   ...THEN LOCK IN:

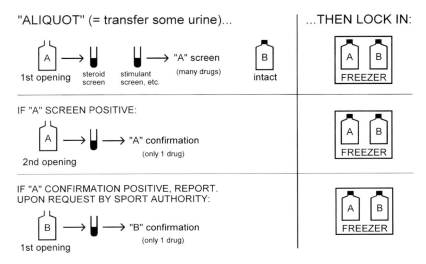

Fig. 1. Typical antidoping laboratory procedure.

steroids), but chemically different between classes, the best conditions for extraction and detection tend to be the same within a class, but different between classes. Typically, laboratories conduct one stimulant screen, one or two steroid screens, one diuretic screen, and so forth on each sample in a batch of test tubes; each test tube represents one athlete. The batch also includes quality-control test tubes.

If the screening data contain any indication that a drug might be present, a fresh portion (aliquot) of the "A" sample undergoes a confirmation attempt. Although a screen collects a little bit of data on each of numerous target compounds, to see if any might be present, a confirmation collects a lot of data on only the suspected compound.

Typically, the time elapsed between receiving the samples at the laboratory and reporting results on the "A" samples (turn-around time) is 1 to 2 weeks for year-round testing, and it can be as short as 24 hours for negative "A" results during major events. "A" confirmations take longer. Results are needed as soon as possible when the world is watching and athletes compete more than once, because if they used drugs, they should be removed from competition.

If the "A" sample analysis confirms the presence of a drug, the laboratory reports to the antidoping program its finding in the sample, identified only by code number—the only identification known to the laboratory. The athlete is notified and has the right to come to the laboratory or send a representative of his or her choice to witness the "B" confirmation. After verification of identity, the witness examines the "B" sample exactly as it was last seen by the athlete when it originally was sealed for shipment to the laboratory; paperwork is filled out and signed. The witness may then observe the "B" confirmation, which takes 2 to 3 days, depending on the drug. Some witnesses choose to watch the process; others choose to leave before the laboratory work begins. After completion and conclusion, the laboratory reports the result of the "B" confirmation to the antidoping program. What remains of positive samples is securely frozen for the length of time that meets applicable regulatory and contractual requirements. Typically, negative samples are disposed of sooner. Disposal is the last entry for each sample's chain of custody documentation.

Main analytical techniques

The goal of this article is to cover key points without being exhaustive and to focus on urine analysis and data interpretation. The laboratories' job is to detect hundreds of substances. Table 1 shows common technologies. The choice of technology is determined primarily by chemical characteristics (eg, solubility in water or organic solvents, volatility, thermolability, polarity) and secondarily by logistics (eg, resident expertise, staff or instrumentation, capacity and throughput in different laboratory sections). Many substances are detected routinely by more than one approach [5,8].

Sample preparation

The work-up ranges from 1 hour to 1 day, depending on the screen. Because metabolism attaches sugars (conjugates) to some drugs (eg, anabolic steroids), the sugars need to be cleaved (deconjugated) using an enzyme (eg, β-glucuronidase) or an acid for some incubation time. The freed drugs that are still too polar and involatile to be vaporized for analysis need to be derivatized, or reacted with chemicals that will "cap" their polar functional groups (eg, to convert hydroxyl groups into trimethylsilyl ether groups in the case of anabolic steroid screening).

Analysis

Chromatography

Chromatography is an analytical chemistry technique used to separate (resolve) the chemical compounds in a mixture. Gas chromatography (GC) is done in the gas phase. A gas chromatograph has three parts: a sample introduction system (injector), an oven containing a chromatography column to achieve separation, and a detector. Typically, a microliter of liquid urine extract is automatically injected into the injector, a chamber at a high temperature. The sample is vaporized and swept along a hair-thin glass tube (capillary column, many meters long, flexible enough to be rolled up in a coil) by a carrier gas (mobile phase), such as helium. Different compounds travel at different speeds because of the differences in boiling point,

Table 1
Screening technologies for classes of prohibited substances and methods

From WADA 2007 prohibited list	Urine screening technology					
	IA	GC	GC-MS	LC-MS or LC-MS-MS	Miscellaneous	IEF
Substances and methods prohibited at all times (in and out of competition)						
Prohibited substances						
Anabolic agents (anabolic steroids)			X	X		
Hormones	hCG, LH					EPO
β-2-agonists			X			
Antiestrogens			X			
Diuretics and other masking agents			X	X		
Prohibited methods						
Enhancement of oxygen transfer			HES, RSR-13		HES dextran by biochemical analyzer	HBOCs
Chemical and physical manipulation						
Gene doping	No urine test					
Substances and methods prohibited in competition						
Stimulants		X				
Narcotics		X				
Cannabinoids	X		X			
Glucocorticosteroids				X		
Substances prohibited in particular sports						
Alcohol					Dipstick or GC	
Beta-blockers			X	X		

polarity, and relative solubility in the carrier gas versus the coating of the inner wall of the column (stationary phase). The compounds emerge from the column outlet at different times after injection (the chromatographic retention time)—separated from each other. Under identical operating conditions, the retention time is characteristic of each chemical compound. If two compounds have the same retention time, they may be identical (eg, testosterone). If two compounds have different retention times, they certainly are different (eg, testosterone and methyltestosterone). Matching retention times between an unknown and a reference standard is one element of identification.

A graph of the amount of substance as a function of the retention time is a chromatogram (Fig. 2A) [9]. Two common GC detectors in antidoping laboratories are the nitrogen-phosphorus detector (NPD) and the mass spectrometer. The NPD detector is ideal for detecting nitrogen-containing compounds, such as stimulants.

Mass spectrometry

Mass spectrometry (MS) is an analytical chemistry technique used for structure elucidation of unknowns or identification of known compounds. A mass spectrometer has three parts: an ion source where the compound is ionized to form a molecular ion and fragmented into smaller ions; a mass filter that separates ions by mass-to-charge ratio (m/z); and a detector. The graph of ion abundance as a function of m/z is a mass spectrum. In Figure 2B, the molecular ion is 360 and significant ions are 345 and 143 (largest = base peak = 100%). The fragmentation pattern is determined by weak bonds and other physicochemical characteristics; therefore, fragmentation is reproducible and characteristic of the molecular structure, and the mass spectrum is like a fingerprint of the compound. Matching mass spectra between an unknown and a reference standard is another element of identification. Significant ions are so characteristic that matching only three ions (eg, 143, 345, 360) and their percent abundance relative to the most intense of the three (eg, 143) has long been widely accepted as proof of chemical identification.

Gas chromatography-mass spectrometry

Gas chromatography-mass spectrometry (GC-MS) is the technique that is used most widely in antidoping labs. The GC effluent enters the mass spectrometer continuously, and the mass spectrometer continuously records roughly one mass spectrum (scan) per second. There are two main modes of MS operation: the full-scan mode and the selected ion monitoring (SIM) mode (see Fig. 2). In the full-scan mode, the mass spectrometer records the whole mass spectrum (from m/z 70 to 400), monitoring hundreds of ions. In the SIM mode, only selected ions are monitored (eg, 143, 345, 360); therefore, a longer time is spent recording each ion. In physics, signal strength (signal-to-noise ratio) increases with the time spent collecting data. Therefore, on

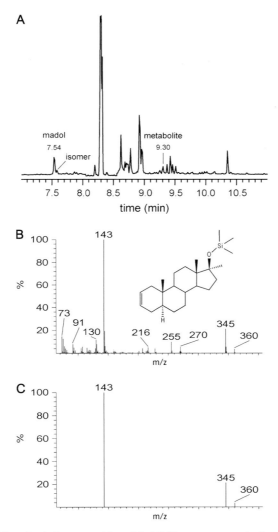

Fig. 2. GC-MS data for designer steroid madol. (*A*) Chromatogram; the isomer differs only by
the position of the double bond. (*B*) Full scan. (*C*) SIM scan.

the same instrument SIM is more sensitive than full scan; it can detect smaller
amounts of drug. Other types of MS that are more sensitive include high-resolution MS, tandem MS, and ion traps. High-resolution MS is designed to
measure m/z not only to the nearest unit or decimal, but out to several
more decimals. This makes it possible to mathematically deduce the molecular formula (how many carbon, hydrogen, oxygen, and other atoms it contains); the more decimals, the fewer combinations of atoms fit, the
narrower the possibilities. High-resolution MS instruments happen to be

inherently more sensitive. Tandem MS instruments have two mass spectrometers back to back. The first one can be used to select only one ion, the precursor ion, which can be the molecular ion. The second mass spectrometer monitors only one (or at most a few) characteristic fragmentations (transitions to product ions). This is called the multiple reaction monitoring or selected reaction monitoring mode. (Alternatively, the first mass spectrometer can be used to select only the molecular ion and the second mass spectrometer can be used to record a full scan.) Tandem MS is more sensitive because it is blind to interferences. Unlike all of the above MS types, which let all ions formed continually escape from the ion source, ion traps trap all ions until they are released, one m/z at a time, to determine their abundance.

Liquid chromatography

Whereas GC is done in the gas phase, liquid chromatography (LC) is done in the liquid phase. This is a crucial difference because it works for thermolabile compounds (destroyed by GC) and polar compounds (cannot be vaporized). The separation principles are the same. A typical high-pressure or high-performance LC (HPLC) column is a steel tube the size of a fat marker pen, packed with microbeads on the surface of which is the stationary phase. The mobile phase is a liquid solvent, often a mixture whose composition is programmed to change during the run (gradient elution).

Two common HPLC detectors are the diode-array detector (DAD) and the mass spectrometer. The DAD monitors UV absorption over a range of wavelengths or at selected wavelengths; it detects only those compounds that absorb UV light. When the HPLC is connected to an MS, the instrument is called LC-MS. The most advanced type of LC-MS can do tandem MS by one of several choices of conceptual and hardware approaches. It is called LC-MS-MS or LC-tandem MS.

For a given class of drugs, such as diuretics (Fig. 3), the LC-tandem MS screen is far superior to the GC-MS screen. Sample preparation time can be well less than 1 hour, down from a full day's work, because unlike GC, LC does not require the removal of water or salts, deconjugation or derivatization. Typically, the instrumental analysis run-time is two to three times shorter, well under 10 minutes per sample, because LC-MS-MS is blind to interferences; therefore, chromatographic resolution is not required, and LC run times can be shortened.

Drug identification

Except for proteins, such as EPO, most prohibited drugs are identified by GC-MS, the workhorse of doping-control laboratories. LC-MS is used increasingly for diuretics, some anabolic steroids, and corticosteroids. Doping-control scientists identify a substance, in the laboratory and in court, by matching chromatographic retention time and mass spectra between unknown and standard. They need an authentic reference standard—a sample of the substance, certified to be correct. The standard may be a white

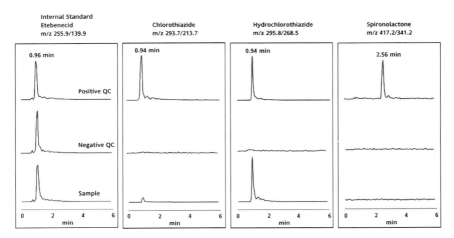

Fig. 3. Example of diuretic screen LC-MS-MS data. Top row: positive quality control (QC) urine spiked with diuretics chlorothiazide, hydrochlorothiazide, and spironolactone. Middle row: negative quality control urine. Bottom row: unknown urine sample. The internal standard (etebenecid) is added to each sample and control during work-up; detecting it shows that the assay performed as expected. Detecting the diuretics spiked into the positive control confirms this. The sample screens positive for hydrochlorothiazide.

powder or an excretion urine from a volunteer who took the drug. Chromatography coupled with MS makes it possible to identify not just drug classes, but specific chemicals, with absolute certainty.

Pharmaceuticals include some synthetic compounds that do not occur naturally (eg, the anabolic steroid stanozolol) and some that do (eg, testosterone). Unfortunately, GC-MS and LC-MS cannot distinguish natural, endogenous testosterone from pharmaceutical, exogenous testosterone; however, normal human urine samples contain a testosterone isomer with no known function, epitestosterone. The urinary ratio of testosterone to epitestosterone (T/E ratio) is roughly 1:1 in most normal men, and it increases upon testosterone administration. Since the 1984 Olympics, the T/E ratio has been used to screen for testosterone use. Adverse analytical findings are defined by a T/E cut-off, which currently is 4. The two problems with any cut-off are that rare, drug-free individuals might have a naturally elevated T/E and that T/E may never exceed the cut-off in some users, either because their T/E is not responsive to administration or because they use small doses and titrate themselves. To distinguish users from nonusers, longitudinal profiling consists of plotting T/E and other urinary androgen parameters over time, expecting stability for nonusers and a spike for users. In the 1990s a new approach was introduced: isotope ratio MS (IRMS) [10].

Isotope ratio mass spectrometry or carbon isotope ratio

It so happens that there is a measurable difference in carbon-13 content between endogenous and pharmaceutical testosterone. Most carbon atoms in nature are carbon-12, with a nucleus containing six protons and six neutrons. Radiocarbon dating relies on the rare carbon-14, an unstable, radioactive isotope, with a nucleus containing six protons and eight neutrons, which decays over time. Between the two is carbon-13, a stable isotope with six protons and seven neutrons. Roughly 1.1% of carbon in nature is carbon-13. Pharmaceutical testosterone contains a few parts per thousand less carbon-13 than does natural testosterone. This is because they arise from biosynthetic pathways that are sufficiently different. Humans make endogenous testosterone from cholesterol, itself made from acetate or coming from the diet. Pharmaceutical companies make testosterone by semisynthesis from plant sterols. All carbon in living beings is ultimately derived from atmospheric carbon dioxide (CO_2), fixed in plants by photosynthesis. Different plants make the first multicarbon intermediates and downstream biosynthetic compounds differently. Animals eat plants, humans eat plants and animals, and we are what we eat. At every biosynthetic step, carbon-13 is left behind. This is because of the isotopic effect: chemical reactions go faster with lighter compounds; the molecule with a carbon-12 reacts sooner than the molecule with a carbon-13 instead. Because the pathways from atmospheric CO_2 to endogenous or pharmaceutical testosterone are different enough, carbon-13 is depleted to different extents; the difference happens to be measurable.

The technique used to make the measurement is GC-combustion-IRMS (GC-C-IRMS). Before application to doping control, it had long been used to detect the fraudulent substitution of synthetic compounds in place of natural compounds in the food, flavor, and fragrance industries. The anabolic steroids are extracted from urine and separated by GC. The separated testosterone enters the pencil-size combustion oven where it is pyrolyzed. Every carbon atom in the molecule is converted to CO_2, and every hydrogen atom is converted to water (H_2O). The water is scrubbed out and only the CO_2 enters the IRMS. This type of MS measures only three m/z: 44 for $^{12}C^{16}O_2$, and 45 and 46 for variants containing carbon-13, oxygen-17, or oxygen-18. From the relative abundances, the instrument software calculates the $\delta^{13}C$ (delta) value. It reflects the $^{13}C/^{12}C$ ratio, but it actually is the difference between the $^{13}C/^{12}C$ ratio of the sample and that of an international standard. The units are ‰ (per mil). By definition, the delta value of the international standard is 0‰. Examples of values are −24‰ for natural testosterone and −29‰ for pharmaceutical testosterone. The values are negative because both compounds contain less carbon-13 than the international standard: 29 fewer parts per thousand for the pharmaceutical testosterone.

After exogenous testosterone administration, the delta values of urinary testosterone metabolites become more negative (Fig. 4). In contrast, the delta values of testosterone precursors, or of endogenous steroids not involved in testosterone metabolism, remain unchanged; therefore, they can be used as endogenous reference compounds. A gap in delta value between testosterone or its metabolites and an endogenous reference compound indicates the use of

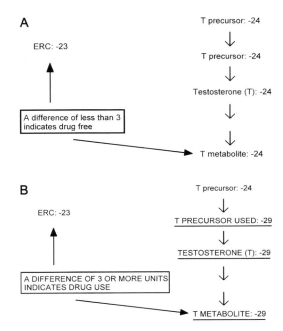

Fig. 4. (*A, B*) How an IRMS test detects doping. A testosterone (T) precursor is metabolized to another T precursor, which is metabolized to T, which undergoes one or more metabolism steps to a T metabolite. Endogenous reference compound (ERC), is a steroid not involved in T metabolism; therefore, it remains unaffected by the administration of pharmaceutical, exogenous T, or of its precursors.

testosterone or of any steroid in its metabolism. If the difference between the delta values of one metabolite and the endogenous reference compound is three delta units or more, the WADA requirement for reporting an adverse analytical finding has been met [11]. The power of this approach is that it can detect the use of not only testosterone itself, but also of any one of many testosterone precursors and metabolites. The second advantage is that it is not affected by factors that might influence baseline delta values. For example, diet influences the carbon-13 content of endogenous steroids—all of them to a similar extent. Although interpreting vastly different delta values from one individual to the next might be difficult, a difference in delta values between a testosterone metabolite and an endogenous reference compound clearly reveals drug use. In short, the approach compensates for individual variability. The third advantage is that it does not require identifying or even knowing what exact compound was taken.

IRMS testing has been applied to various testosterone precursors, testosterone metabolites, and endogenous reference compounds. It is currently done for samples with T/E greater than 4 or on request by the sports authority.

Isoelectric focusing

Isoelectric focusing (IEF) is used to detect recombinant EPO in the urine EPO test [12–14]. Historically, the EPO test at the Olympics (2000 to 2006) was done on paired blood and urine samples collected simultaneously. The blood test is an indirect test because it does not detect the presence of recombinant EPO. Instead, it measures multiple parameters (eg, hemoglobin, hematocrit, percentage of reticulocytes) and calculates a score that indicates whether the individual is on or recently off recombinant EPO [15]. Since 2002, EPO tests done by United States sports authorities have included only the urine test, a direct test that identifies recombinant EPO. EPO tests are done on only some of all of the urine samples, upon request by the sports authority.

Endogenous human EPO is a glycoprotein with a known amino acid sequence and glycosylation pattern. More precisely, it consists of a family of isoforms (molecules that differ only by their degrees of glycosylation). As a result, the pH at which each isoform bears as many negative charges as positive charges (isoelectric point or PI) is different.

Recombinant human EPO differs from endogenous human EPO only by its overall glycosylation pattern (ie, it consists of a different family of isoforms). The difference in overall pattern of isoforms allows differentiation between recombinant and endogenous human EPO.

The urine EPO test, also known as the French test or the IEF test, consists of four steps: sample preparation, IEF, double blotting, and visualization. Sample preparation concentrates EPO by multiple ultrafiltrations that leave the proteins of desired molecular weight in the filtration "retentate."

Next, the retentate is deposited on a gel with an embedded pH gradient, and a current is applied to achieve electrophoretic separation of the isoforms (IEF). Unknown samples, reference standards, and known positive and negative quality controls are normally run on each gel. Each sample, standard, or control spreads out in its own "lane." Each isoform is charged; therefore, it migrates in the electrical field until it reaches the distance on the gel at which the pH is equal to its PI. There the isoform is electrically neutral so it stops migrating. Its position or distance up the gel is key, and the goal of the remaining steps is to visualize it.

The first blotting step transfers all proteins (erythropoietic and other) to a first membrane. The membrane is incubated with antibodies specific to erythropoietic proteins. The second blot transfers only these specific antibodies to the second membrane, thus transferring the isoform pattern, but leaving behind all proteins, including some that otherwise would obscure the final image.

Visualization is based on chemiluminescence; it involves incubation with a second antibody that binds to the first antibody and a chemical reaction that emits light. The image (electropherogram) is captured with a special digital camera. All steps use commonplace molecular biology techniques. The electropherogram contains one lane per sample, standard, or quality control sample (Fig. 5). In each lane, the isoform pattern consists of bands. The pattern (number of bands, positions, relative intensities) allows identification.

In common language, a negative EPO test often is discussed as if it reflects the absence of EPO, but of course what it means is that there was no recombinant erythropoietic protein in the urine sample, which normally would (hopefully!) contain natural, endogenous EPO.

Blood tests

Blood screening [5] is done at the Olympics, but not in the main United States sports drug-testing programs. At the 2004 Athens Olympics, whole blood was tested by cytometry to detect blood transfusions. Serum was tested by LC-MS-MS to detect hemoglobin-based oxygen carriers and by immunoassay to detect recombinant human growth hormone (GH). Natural GH is a family of isoforms, including a major one of 22 kd (22,000 atomic mass units) and some non–22-kd isoforms, whereas recombinant GH is 100% 22-kd isoforms. Administration of recombinant GH suppresses endogenous GH production. The current approach to recombinant GH detection in serum is based on estimating the ratio of the 22-kd isoform to non–22-kd isoforms by immunoassay; it can detect administration for 3 hours after the last dose [16]. The test was conducted at the 2006 Winter Games in Torino as well. No adverse analytical findings were reported. This test can be implemented more widely as soon as reagents can be manufactured in sufficient quantities [17].

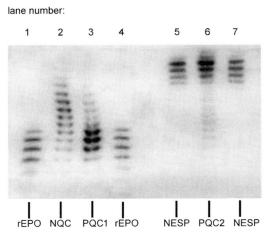

Fig. 5. EPO test result. Lane number and content: 1 & 4: rEPO = recombinant EPO (rEPO), pure standard; 2: NQC = negative quality control = research subject urine before rEPO administration; 3: PQC1 = positive quality control 1 = research subject urine after rEPO administration; 5 & 7: NESP = darbepoetin = long-lasting rEPO, pure standard; 6: PQC2 = positive quality control 2 = urine from different research subject after NESP administration.

Laboratory report interpretation

The laboratory urine drug test can determine what substance is present in the urine sample, not the brand, formulation, route of administration, dose, or how long before urine collection the drug was taken. Reasons why a urine drug test is negative include the drug is not prohibited by this program; the drug was never used; the drug was used long enough ago to have been eliminated completely; the drug is present below the cut-off; the drug is present below the limit of detection of the test; the drug is a prohibited (designer) drug that the laboratory does not look for; the sample was manipulated; and the sample was not real urine. The latter can be revealed by steroid screen data devoid of natural steroids in cases that would be missed by commercial adulteration tests and dipsticks.

Many factors determine test retrospectivity (Table 2), or how long after the end of administration the test can detect the drug in urine: among them are the dose, body burden, elimination pharmacokinetics, and test sensitivity. Anabolic steroids can be detected for as little as only a few days or as long as many months after the user stops taking them, depending on the type used (eg, short-acting pill or long-acting oily injection), how much was used, and for how long. In addition, some steroids are easier to detect than others because of chemical differences. Individuals who have been in a drug-testing program for some time are less likely to use long-acting, easy-to-detect steroids.

The test result on a follow-up sample collected some time after an initial, positive sample needs to be interpreted in light of the above. If the follow-up test is positive for the same drug, it may be because the drug was not completely eliminated yet or because the athlete used the drug again in the meantime. Comparing the laboratory data from both tests may or may not provide an indication of which is the case. The follow-up test is expected to be negative if the drug was eliminated completely. This is why a negative follow-up test is not relevant to determining the accuracy or inaccuracy of a positive result on a sample collected previously. Conversely, a negative follow-up test is a valid check that the athlete has stopped using the drug.

Table 2
Urine drug test retrospectivity

Prohibited drugs	Period of detectability after last dose
Stimulants	A few hours to a few days
Anabolic steroids	From a few days (short-acting, water soluble, small doses) to many months (long-acting oily injection, large doses for a long time)
Diuretics	A few hours to a few days
Marijuana	Some weeks
rEPO	A few days

Drug users who expect to be tested at events try to time their discontinuation to pass the test; this is why no-notice, out-of-competition testing was implemented in the 1980s. In the early 2000s, United States track and field athlete Kelli White passed 17 drug tests while on steroids (tetrahydrogestrinone [THG], testosterone), stimulants (modafinil), and EPO before she was caught on modafinil, then confessed to having used the whole regimen [18]. THG was not found in her samples because laboratories were still blind to this designer steroid (used only to beat the test). Testosterone use was not detected because she masked it by taking epitestosterone as well; because her T/E never exceeded the cut-off, it never triggered IRMS analysis, which would have detected exogenous testosterone. Modafinil was first targeted and found by the French WADA-accredited laboratory; her EPO use was not detected because sprinters' samples were not tested for EPO yet.

It is said that the test is blind to designer steroids, because the test is targeted and finds only what it looks for. Typically, WADA-accredited laboratories screen for most anabolic steroids by GC-MS in the more sensitive SIM mode, monitoring only a few ions per target compound (eg, an ion of 415 atomic mass units). A designer steroid could differ from a known one by only two extra hydrogens, give an ion of 417 atomic mass units upon fragmentation, and escape detection because the test monitors 415, not 417. Or the designer steroid could fragment to ions that happen to be monitored, in which case data readers would see suspicious signals and investigate further. The first reported designer steroid (norbolethone) [19] was a pharmaceutical abandoned decades before, during clinical trials. It resurfaced upon further investigation of an athlete's urine sample devoid of normal endogenous androgens, a telltale sign of endocrine suppression, which is expected after androgen administration because of negative feedback. The second designer steroid (THG) [20] was discovered because a coach turned in a used syringe. THG simply is not detected in the standard steroid screen, probably because its chemical properties are such that it disintegrates along the way. Different modifications of the screen now allow its detection.

Are the tests accurate? What are the risks of "false positive" or "false negative"? Both phrases can have widely different meanings in common language compared with antidoping jargon. In common language, a "false positive" might be any adverse analytical finding that does not result in a sanction, perhaps because the athlete had a therapeutic use exemption, because a courier's signature was missing on a shipping document, or because the prohibited drug was a supplement contaminant. Supplements are not regulated by the US Food and Drug Administration (FDA); athletes should not only use them at their own risk but question whether they need them to win [21]. A case in which on appeal, an arbitrators' panel had purely legal reasons to exonerate the athlete, might casually be called a "false positive." But for the laboratory, a false positive is only the case in which the laboratory reports the presence of a drug and it is later proven scientifically that the drug was not present.

As for a "false negative," in common language that might be a case where the athlete used a drug but passed the test. This could be because the metabolite was accurately detected just below the cut-off—a perfectly accurate negative result. Other possible explanations for negative results following drug use were listed above.

Handling of results by the sports authority

Based on the laboratory "B" report, the sports authority decides whether to charge the athlete with a doping offense. For USADA, the process includes automatic consideration by a Review Board and the opportunity for the athlete to request an arbitration hearing to contest the sanction [22]. The NCAA protocol includes an appeal process [23]. The laboratory remains involved when additional documentation (administrative or technical), scientific support for the legal team, or testimony is requested.

When doping cases lead to legal activities, the laboratories' decision criteria are reviewed. The WADA criteria for drug identification are not novel; they have long been widely used. GC-MS, LC-MS, and GC-C-IRMS technology were not invented for doping control; instead doping control is merely one of many fields of application.

The days of genuine or alleged inadvertent use being excused are over now that strict liability is enforced. It has room for refinement (lesser penalties) when authorities believe that the athlete made an honest mistake. Sanctions for the athlete's entourage (eg, team physicians) are meted out in more cases.

Antidoping program administrators and attorneys, such as those of USADA, are the third key link in the chain that began with the sample collection team and continued with the laboratory team. They take the drug test result to its final conclusion, carrying the baton over the finish line. They also have gone beyond drug testing by charging athletes in cases involving "non-analytical positives" (ie, evidence of doping that does not include a positive test result).

Testing statistics are available online. In 2000, WADA took over the IOC's annual collection of statistics from worldwide accredited laboratories, including the total number of samples tested per laboratory and number of adverse analytical findings (total per laboratory, per drug worldwide, and per sport worldwide) [24]. USADA posts annual testing statistics and the test history of all United States athletes tested by USADA since its inception in 2000 [25]. The NCAA results since 2001 are online [26].

Current trends

Will antidoping science ever get ahead of the cheats? (Not that we can ever catch every last one.) The pace of medical progress makes doping control an endless escalade in complication and expense. If society wants no performance-enhancing drugs in sports, the prospects for a technological fix for values gone out of line might be dim. This is, in part, because crooked scientists can market new designer drugs overnight with no concern for FDA approval, and some athletes pay good money to be the ones to discover safety and efficacy... or the lack thereof. Meanwhile, antidoping scientists need months or years to develop and validate new tests.

Yet major, recent improvements include the increased commitment of government entities in the United States and in Europe to the fight against doping, the speed at which sports authorities will add a drug to the prohibited list, and the expansion of profiling as a means to detect drug use.

Physicians have long monitored patient biomarkers (eg, blood cholesterol) for preventive purposes. Drug use is expected to affect common clinical test results and additional ones selected for their responsiveness to doping agents. Two examples are how longitudinal T/E profiling helps to spot users and how the absence of endogenous urinary steroids led to the discovery of the designer steroid norbolethone. Extending the review of steroid profiles to all athletes undergoing doping-control tests has not been done yet—although it has long been possible technically because urinary steroid profiles are archived at laboratories, and sports authorities know which bottle numbers represent each athlete. Now that blood collection is more common in sports, more parameters could be added. Several programs in different countries are gearing up to formally and prospectively collect athlete urine and blood profile data. Some of those programs are voluntary, and although they all look similar at first glance, only one of them is all carrots and no sticks: envisioned by Don Catlin [27], it is designed to help clean athletes show the world that they are drug-free, so that when they win they do not have to suffer suspicion of drug use. Beyond public recognition, the program might offer free medical care and nutrition and fitness advice. Deviations from normal variability would be discussed with a trusted health care team. If a deviation had no explanation other than drug use, the athlete merely would be dropped from the program. No athlete would be sanctioned or suspended from competition or kicked off teams or contracts. With no sanctions, the lower risk for legal activities would lower the cost of the program. The central question would be: "What if an anti-doping program rewarded drug-free athletes instead of punishing drug-using athletes?" Could it trigger a shift in culture or is that just a wild hope for a crazy idea?

At the heart of any program is a trusting relationship with health care professionals, something that patients can experience at a young age with their pediatricians, who could be among the most influential people in turning around the culture of drug use in sports.

Summary

Pediatricians or their patients may have to deal with sports-doping control tests and positive results. A substantial international regulatory framework is in place to harmonize sports rules and drug-testing laboratories. In major programs, urine and blood samples are split into an "A" and a "B" sample, and urination is observed directly. Chain of custody paperwork documents who has custody of the samples or where they are locked up, from the moment the bottles are sealed, to their receipt at the laboratory, to the day when they are finally discarded. If an "A" sample screens positive, the finding is confirmed twice before sanctions are considered: by reanalyzing the "A" sample and then analyzing the "B" sample. The main analytical chemistry technologies in doping-control laboratories are GC-MS, LC-MS-MS, IRMS detection of exogenous testosterone use, and IEF detection of recombinant EPO use. The approaches, technologies, and drug identification criteria are not novel; they have long been widely used in other fields. Although every medical advance has a potential for abuse by athletes, overnight and underground, antidoping scientists, who work above board, are slowed by the requirements of testing research, development, and validation. To try to leap ahead of the curve, the newest trend in doping control is the expansion of all elite athletes' profiling by monitoring biomarkers and watching for deviations that may be indicative of drug use.

Acknowledgments

Many thanks to Don Catlin for illuminating discussions, Brian Ahrens for superb assistance with figures, and to Patrick Do, Charles Do, MD, Gary Green, MD, and Richard Hilderbrand, PhD, for editorial advice.

References

[1] The World Anti-Doping Code. The 2007 prohibited list international standard. Available at: http://www.wada-ama.org/rtecontent/document/2007_List_En.pdf. Accessed February 13, 2007.
[2] WADA technical document TD2004MRPL. Minimum required performance limits for detection of prohibited substances. Available at: http://www.wada-ama.org/rtecontent/document/perf_limits_2.pdf. Accessed February 14, 2007.
[3] NCAA banned-drug classes 2006–2007. Available at: http://www1.ncaa.org/membership/ed_outreach/health-safety/drug_testing/banned_drug_classes.pdf. Accessed February 13, 2007.
[4] The World Anti-Doping Code. International standard for laboratories version 4.0. Available at: http://www.wada-ama.org/rtecontent/document/lab_aug_04.pdf. Accessed February 14, 2007.
[5] Tsivou M, Kioukia-Fougia N, Lyris E, et al. An overview of the doping control analysis during the Olympic Games of 2004 in Athens, Greece. Anal Chim Acta 2006;555:1–13.
[6] UCI Cycling Regulations. Part 13 sporting safety and conditions. Available at: http://www.uci.ch/imgArchive/Rules/13con-E.pdf. Accessed February 15, 2007.
[7] Cheating on a drug test. Available at: http://www.drugfreesportcom/insight.asp?VolID=31&;TopicID=7. Accessed February 14, 2007.
[8] Trout GJ, Kazlauskas R. Sports drugs testing—an analyst's perspective. Chem Soc Rev 2004;33:1–13.

[9] Sekera MH, Ahrens B, Chang YC, et al. Another designer steroid: discovery, synthesis, and detection of 'madol' in urine. Rapid Commun Mass Spectrom 2005;19:781–4.

[10] Aguilera R, Chapman TE, Starcevic B, et al. Performance characteristics of a carbon isotope ratio method for detecting doping with testosterone based on urine diols: controls and athletes with elevated testosterone/epitestosterone ratios. Clin Chem 2001;47:292–300.

[11] WADA Technical Document TD2004EAAS Version 1.0. Reporting and evaluation guidance for testosterone, epitestosterone, T/E ratio and other endogenous steroids. Available at: http://www.wada-ama.org/rtecontent/document/end_steroids_aug_04.pdf. Accessed February 13, 2007.

[12] Lasne F, Martin L, Crepin N, et al. Detection of isoelectric profiles of erythropoietin in urine: differentiation of natural and administered recombinant hormones. Anal Biochem 2002;311: 119–26.

[13] Catlin DH, Breidbach A, Elliott S, et al. Comparison of the isoelectric focusing patterns of darbepoetin alfa, recombinant human erythropoietin, and endogenous erythropoietin from human urine. Clin Chem 2002;48:2057–9.

[14] WADA Technical Document TD2004EPO Version 1.0. Harmonization of the method for the identification of epoetin alfa and beta (EPO) and darbepoetin alfa (NESP) by IEF-double blotting and chemiluminescent detection. Available at: http://www.wada-ama.org/rtecontent/document/td2004epo_en.pdf. Accessed February 13, 2007.

[15] Parisotto R, Gore CJ, Emslie KR, et al. A novel method utilising markers of altered erythropoiesis for the detection of recombinant human erythropoietin in athletes. Haematologica 2000;85:564–72.

[16] Wallace JD, Cuneo RC, Bidlingmaier M, et al. Changes in non-22-kilodalton (kDa) isoforms of growth hormone (GH) after administration of 22-kDa recombinant human GH in trained adult males. J Clin Endocrinol Metab 2001;86:1731–7.

[17] Bowers L. Lessons learned from recent doping investigations and athlete cases. In: Doping: the World Anti-Doping Program and the role of medical care providers in doping and anti-doping efforts. Workshop #14, 20 February 2007. Presented at the 59th Annual Meeting of the American Academy of Forensic Scientists. San Antonio (TX).

[18] Testimony of Kelli White, U.S. Olympian, former steroid user, to the U.S. Senate. Available at: http://commerce.senate.gov/hearings/testimony.cfm?id=1511&;wit_id=4276. Accessed February 16, 2007.

[19] Catlin DH, Ahrens BD, Kucherova Y. Detection of norbolethone, an anabolic steroid never marketed, in athletes' urine. Rapid Commun Mass Spectrom 2002;16:1273–5.

[20] Catlin DH, Sekera MH, Ahrens B, et al. Tetrahydrogestrinone: discovery, synthesis, and detection in urine. Rapid Commun Mass Spectrom 2004;18:1245–9.

[21] Can you win without supplements?. Available at: http://www.drugfreesport.com. Accessed February 14, 2007.

[22] USADA protocol for Olympic movement testing. Available at: http://www.usantidoping.org/files/active/what/protocol.pdf. Accessed February 14, 2007.

[23] NCAA Drug-Testing Program 2006–2007. Available at: http://www.ncaa.org/library/sports_sciences/drug_testing_program/2006-07/2006-07_drug_testing_program.pdf. Accessed February 14, 2007.

[24] WADA program statistics. Available at: http://www.wada-ama.org/en/dynamic.ch2?pageCategory.id=328. Accessed February 14, 2007.

[25] USADA testing statistics. Available at: http://www.usantidoping.org/what/stats/. Accessed January 26, 2007.

[26] NCAA drug-testing program overview and results archive. Available at: http://www.ncaa.org/sports_sciences/drugtesting/drug_testing_results_archive.html. Accessed February 14, 2007.

[27] Alexander B. The awful truth about drugs in sports. Outside July 2005;100-108. Available at: http://outside.away.com/outside/features/200507/drugs-in-sports-1.html. Accessed February 16, 2007.

ELSEVIER
SAUNDERS

PEDIATRIC CLINICS
OF NORTH AMERICA

Pediatr Clin N Am 54 (2007) 735–760

Creatine and Other Supplements

Anthony Lattavo, DO[a],*, Andrew Kopperud, MD[b,c],
Peter D. Rogers, MD, MPH, FAAP[c,d]

[a]Department of Medical Education, Grant Medical Center, 285 East State Street,
Suite 670, Columbus, OH 43215-4354, USA
[b]Columbus Children's Hospital, 700 Children's Drive, Columbus, OH 43205, USA
[c]The Ohio State University College of Medicine, Columbus, OH 43210, USA
[d]Section of Adolescent Health, Columbus Children's Hospital, 700 Children's Drive,
Columbus, OH 43205, USA

The dietary supplement industry in the United States is growing rapidly, with annual sales of approximately $18 billion [1]. Ergogenic supplement use (ie, for the purpose of enhancing athletic performance) is increasing among adolescent and collegiate athletes, and the average age of initiation of use is decreasing [2]. In the adolescent population, use is estimated at 24% to 29%, and the likelihood of use increases with increasing physical activity [3]. One large study found that about two thirds of supplement use starts before college, and 9.2% begins before high school [2]. The most common supplements used by collegiate athletes (all sports combined) are as follows (percentage of athletes reporting use in parentheses): protein products (70.4%), creatine (39.6%), amino acids (20.4%), thermogenics/weight loss (5.1%), beta-hydroxy-beta-methylbutyrate (HMB) (1.9%), chromium (1.6%), and others (17.3%) [2]. To provide appropriate recommendations for or against use by individual athletes, the physician working with adolescent and collegiate athletes should be familiar with these most commonly used supplements and be able to locate high-quality information about the multitude of "others."

Athletes obtain information about supplements from a variety of sources, including friends, teammates, coaches, trainers, family members, physicians, dietitians, and the media (including the Internet) [3]. The quality of information provided by many of these sources is poor and biased; highly motivated athletes tend to accept information that promises performance gains and reject information that presents a lack of performance benefit or a risk for adverse effects. Therefore, the physician must avoid the "just say no"

---

* Corresponding author.
  E-mail address: alattavo@columbus.rr.com (A. Lattavo).

doi:10.1016/j.pcl.2007.04.009   *pediatric.theclinics.com*

approach and give sound advice based on scientific data (or lack thereof), educating the athlete in the process [4]. One also must consider that information about efficacy and safety of dietary supplement use in adolescents is scarce compared with such information in adult populations. Pharmacodynamically and pharmacokinetically, the adolescent body may handle and respond to supplements differently than adults, resulting in less predictable ergogenic and adverse effects [3]. Also, athletes of all ages use supplements in an infinite number of combinations. Although the individual agents may be well studied in isolation, there may not be any good scientific information to guide the use of them in combination.

Regulation of dietary supplements

To make appropriate recommendations to athletes regarding dietary supplements, one must have a basic understanding of their definition, classification, and regulatory environment. An understanding of the dietary supplement industry's regulatory environment is enhanced by comparing and contrasting it with that of the prescription drug industry. The notion that the dietary supplement industry is unregulated is a common misconception among health care professionals. Dietary supplements are regulated primarily by the US Food and Drug Administration (FDA), but also by the Federal Trade Commission (FTC); however, supplements are regulated much differently, and much less rigorously, than are the drug products that physicians prescribe every day. The FDA and the FTC cooperate in regulating the dietary supplement industry [5]. The FDA is responsible for product safety and labeling, including label claims and promotional literature at the point of sale [5]. The FTC regulates the advertising of dietary supplements, including print and broadcast advertisements, infomercials, catalogs, and Internet Web sites [5]. The Dietary Supplements Health and Education Act of 1994 (DSHEA) is the preeminent legislation that comprehensively defines and governs dietary supplements in the United States [6]. Originally, the DSHEA was intended to facilitate greater consumer access to dietary supplements that may have positive health benefits; in the process, it weakened the FDA's authority over the supplement market [7].

Definition and classification

Dietary supplements are classified as a subcategory of "foods" and have a specific definition:

A product (other than tobacco) that is intended to supplement the diet that bears or contains one or more of the following dietary ingredients: a vitamin, a mineral, an herb or other botanical, an amino acid, a dietary substance for use by man to supplement the diet by increasing the total daily intake, or a concentrate, metabolite, constituent, extract, or combinations of these ingredients

Intended for ingestion in pill, capsule, tablet, or liquid form

Not represented for use as a conventional food or as the sole item of a meal or diet

Labeled as a "dietary supplement" [6]

Product approval and assurance of safety

In contrast to drugs, supplements have much less stringent requirements for new product approval. For drug products, "premarket approval" is required, in which the FDA requires extensive research data demonstrating that a drug's health benefits outweigh its risks before it approves the product for sale [8]. In general, there is no premarket approval process for dietary supplements (the exception being supplements that contain "new dietary ingredients"; see later discussion). To market a supplement, the manufacturer does not have to provide the FDA with any efficacy data per se, although the manufacturer is responsible for the accuracy of claims it makes concerning the product [9]. Regarding safety, if the supplement's ingredients were marketed in the United States before the passage of the DSHEA, then the product is presumed to be safe, and the manufacturer can market the product without providing safety data or even notifying the FDA [9,10]. However, if the supplement contains a "new dietary ingredient" (ie, one not marketed before passage of the DSHEA), it is presumed to be unsafe, and the manufacturer must provide the FDA with safety data at least 75 days before marketing the product [9,11,12]. The FDA reviews this evidence and decides whether to take action to prevent the product from reaching the market [11]. The FDA has been stringent with new dietary ingredients, accepting fewer than 30% of new dietary ingredient submissions [12]. This process is conceptually similar to the process of premarket approval for drug products, although there is an important distinction. When considering a new drug application, the FDA performs a "risk/benefit" analysis to determine whether it is adequately safe for use; however, the FDA is not required to assess a new dietary ingredient's efficacy when it decides whether there is reasonable assurance of safety to permit it to be marketed [9]. This results in a great degree of subjectivity in this determination. "Adequate safety" can only truly be determined when the degree of potential benefit is known and considered. For the many dietary supplements that have little or no evidence of significant benefit, it is difficult to determine whether there is "adequate safety" to justify use.

Once on the market, the manufacturer (not the FDA) is responsible for assuring the supplement's safety, and the lack of diligence by manufacturers in investigating side effects and safety issues has been criticized [4,10]. At this point, the FDA can act against a product only if it poses a significant health threat. In such situations, the FDA has the burden of proving that the use of a supplement, as recommended on the label, is unsafe [8–10,13]. Then, the US Secretary of Health and Human Services has the authority to order the supplement removed from the market; however, before doing so, the government is required to convene hearings to review the evidence for taking such a measure, potentially delaying necessary action [5]. In recent years, the FDA has taken action in this manner in removing several supplements from the market, including ephedra and androstenedione.

Product labeling

Supplement product labeling has specific regulations, including (1) information that must be presented on the label (eg, a statement identifying the product as a dietary supplement with a list of ingredients present in "significant amounts" and their quantities); (2) information that needs not be presented (eg, disclosure of ingredients not present in "significant amounts"); and (3) claims that may be made about the product on its label and in its package [6]. Several types of claims can be made about supplements. With ergogenic supplements, the most pertinent of these are structure/function claims, which are statements describing the effect of a supplement on the structure or function of the body [14]. This type of claim also may describe a mechanism by which the supplement acts to maintain such structure or function [8]. Supplements with structure/function claims are not subject to premarket review by the FDA, and a disclosure must be present on the label, stating that the FDA has not evaluated the claim and that the product is not intended to diagnose, treat, cure, or prevent any disease [8,14]. The manufacturer is responsible for the truthfulness of its claims, and, although the DSHEA requires the manufacturer to have evidence to support them, there is no requirement that such evidence be provided to the FDA for its review before marketing the product [8,10]. Turner and colleagues [8] questioned the degree to which the FDA has enforced misleading claims regulations, stating that because of its limited resources it has made product safety a higher priority. Their article is an excellent review of label claims for supplements.

Quality assurance and standardization

The issues of quality of the manufacturing process and product standardization raise concern as well. The FDA has the authority to establish current "good manufacturing practices" (GMPs) that are specific for dietary supplements, but it has not done so [15]. The current GMPs for supplements are the same as those for conventional food products, and the degree of enforcement is questionable [7]. The FDA does not inspect manufacturing facilities, and it does not routinely perform premarket or after-market testing of dietary supplements [11]. Product testing is done only if an adverse event occurs that triggers concern about safety [10]. The manufacturer is responsible for ensuring standardization and reliability [16]. Compliance with these requirements is clearly suboptimal, as numerous studies have analyzed individual supplements and found them to contain ingredient quantities inconsistent with quantities listed on the label (usually less than the stated amount, sometimes containing none of the stated ingredients, and sometimes even containing ingredients not listed on the label, including substances that would cause positive drug tests for banned substances) [17–21]. In 2001, Green and colleagues [19] tested 12 different androgen precursor supplement brands (legal at the time but currently banned by most sporting organizations) purchased from retail stores in Los Angeles, California; 11 were mislabeled according to DSHEA requirements. Most supplements contained less than the stated amount, but one of them contained 10 mg of testosterone, an illegal anabolic steroid. Baume and colleagues [18] tested 103 legal supplements obtained from Web sites in Europe and in America; 18% were contaminated with substances not disclosed on the label. Most of the contaminated supplements were androgen precursors, but one was a creatine supplement contaminated with several androgen precursors that have been known to cause positive urine tests for metabolites of nandrolone, a banned anabolic steroid. One "mental enhancer" stated to contain caffeine was found to contain an androgen precursor. Significant dose-to-dose variability also has been found within individual supplement packages [22]. Because of these findings, a supplement's product labeling cannot be relied upon to ascertain the actual ingredient content, especially when the stakes are high for elite athletes [18]. From a scientific standpoint, the lack of uniformity makes supplements difficult to study [4]. To the athlete, these findings are important for two reasons. First, if a supplement does not contain the stated amount of an ergogenic ingredient, the athlete may lose the potential benefit of taking it. Second, athletes subject to drug testing who test positive for banned substances, are—in most jurisdictions—judged according to the "strict liability" principle, which holds the athlete responsible for what is found in his/her body, regardless of whether the athlete knowingly ingested the banned substance [21,23].

Out of the lack of standardization and reliability have emerged several independent agencies (eg, ConsumerLab.com, National Sanitation Foundation International, and the U.S. Pharmacopeia's Dietary Supplement Verification Program) that perform testing of supplements' quality and integrity [24–26]. They perform initial supplement analysis and random off-the-shelf testing of supplements at the manufacturer's request and expense, in exchange providing a seal of approval on the label if the product meets its standards. ConsumerLab.com provides its findings to paid subscribers on its Web site. These are several means by which athletes can verify the quality and integrity of the products that they are considering using.

Commentary

Although the DSHEA established regulations for the marketing of dietary supplements, manufacturers' compliance with regulations and the

FDA's enforcement of them have been seriously questioned [5,16]. Since the passage of the DSHEA, the regulatory environment has evolved as the legislation has been interpreted, and this process will continue in the future. There is some evidence that the FDA is trying to regain more control over the dietary supplement industry [7]. Wollschlaeger [5] contended that the FDA and FTC have sufficient legislative authority to provide optimal consumer protection from unsafe products and untruthful claims and advertising, and that rather than establish new rules and regulations, adequate funding and other resources should be provided to the FDA and FTC for them to function as legally intended in the dietary supplement arena.

Creatine

Prevalence of use

Although creatine was discovered more than 100 years ago, and its use as a performance-enhancing supplement has been occurring for some time, there have been few studies on the frequency of use and patterns of use until recent years, particularly among adolescents. One of the first large-scale studies of creatine use was performed by the National Collegiate Athletic Association (NCAA) in 1997. The study, which surveyed nearly 14,000 athletes from Division I, II, and III, reported that 32% of those surveyed had used creatine in the last 12 months [27]. Since that time there have been multiple other studies documenting the prevalence of creatine use among professional and collegiate athletes.

Given the high frequency of creatine use among professional and collegiate athletes, there has been legitimate concern regarding the use of creatine by adolescent athletes. Smith and Dahm [28] were among the first to report findings based primarily on adolescent athletes in 2000. Their study, although small, showed that 8.2% of the athletes surveyed had ever used creatine, and 52% of those were using it at the time of the survey. Users in their sample were composed primarily (89%) of athletes who played football, hockey, or basketball. Even more concerning, however, was the fact that the primary source of information on creatine was their friends (74%). Subsequently, 55% of their athletes did not know the dose of creatine they were taking, and another 23% reported taking a dose higher than the recommended maintenance dose.

Given the significance of these findings, there has been other research in this area. A 2001 study of 674 high school athletes in Tennessee and Georgia reported that 16% of the athletes surveyed used creatine. Twenty-three percent of the boys in the study used creatine, and 2% of the girls used it. The study also found that creatine use tended to increase with age and grade. In line with the previous study, 70% of the athletes surveyed reported taking excessive amounts of creatine as a maintenance dose [29]. Another slightly larger study at about the same time showed that 5.6% of athletes surveyed in a suburban New York population admitted to taking creatine (8.8% of boys and 1.8% of girls). In this study, creatine was used most commonly by athletes who participated in gymnastics, hockey, wrestling, football, and lacrosse. This study also showed an increase in creatine use with an increase in grade in school, although it did show use as early as sixth grade [30]. Finally, a 2001 study of Wisconsin high school football players showed that 30% were using creatine, including more than 50% of the seniors surveyed [31].

These first studies were performed primarily using young athletes as a population; however, more recent studies also showed significant creatine use among all adolescents. A 2003 study of 333 Canadian adolescents reported that 5.3% of those surveyed reported using creatine; those who reported using creatine reported an average of 23 hours per week of physical activity versus 12.2 hours for those who did not report creatine use. The latter numbers, however, were not significant based on the power of their study [32]. A subsequent 2005 study of dietary supplement use in adolescents showed that 4.7% of adolescents reported ever using creatine [33]. A recent large-scale study of 15,000 adolescents showed that 8% of adolescents reported using a legal performance-enhancing supplement in the past year; youth participating in sports were about 1.5 times more likely to have done so [34].

Mechanism of action

Although the use of creatine as a performance-enhancing substance seems to be a new phenomenon, creatine originally was described in the 1830s by Chevreul; it has undergone extensive study since that time. Creatine is a nonessential amino acid that is formed in the liver by a two-step process from arginine and glycine; it also is found in varying amounts in different meats [35,36]. Creatine is taken up by muscle cells by way of a sodium-dependent transporter [36]. Once in the cells, creatine is believed to have multiple functions through which supplementation may enhance exercise performance. All of these major functions center around the following reaction of the enzyme creatine kinase:

$$MgADP^- + PCr^{2-} + H^+ \leftrightarrow MgATP^{2-} + Cr$$

Creatine then gives rise to five major functions within skeletal muscle cells [37].

The first of these functions of the "phosphocreatine system" is to serve as a "temporal energy buffer" within the cell. The main purpose is the direct rephosphorylation of ATP from phosphocreatine as a means of "buffering" against changes in ATP during short-duration exercise [36]. This is corroborated by the fact that there seems to be little difference in total cell ATP in muscle cells whether they are contracted or relaxed [38]. In addition to being an acute energy buffer for the regeneration of ATP within the cell, it is generally accepted that the phosphocreatine system serves as a transport system for energy between sites of energy production and sites of energy use. This is supported most significantly by a surprising amount of evidence regarding the compartmentation of creatine kinase isoenzymes within the cell [37].

Not only does the phosphocreatine system give cells a specialized system of energy buffer and energy transport, it serves three other biochemical functions within the cell. The first of these is to buffer against an increase in intracellular ADP, which prevents inhibition of ATP-dependent processes and prevents a net loss of adenine nucleotide pools by way of adenylate kinase [37,39]. The reaction also helps to prevent intracellular acidosis during exercise by consuming hydrogen ions [36]. Finally, the system plays an important role in providing an appropriate ATP/ADP ratio in localized areas of the cell. For example, in muscle cells, the action of creatine kinase allows for a larger amount of ATP at the myofibril, while providing a higher amount of ADP at the mitochondria, which can then be rephosphorylated to ATP by way of oxidative phosphorylation [37].

Although the physiologic effects of creatine within the body are important and likely play a vital role in the effectiveness of creatine as a performance-enhancing substance, there has been some evidence that ingestion of exogenous creatine may have other effects within the cell. First of all, it is believed that ingestion of creatine and uptake into cells increases water intake into the cells by osmotic action [40]. Secondary to this, there seems to be an increase in body mass after ingestion of creatine, especially in young, healthy men [36]. It also is theorized that the increase in intracellular water may have the effect of decreasing the breakdown of protein within the cell and possibly also increasing protein synthesis within the cell [41].

Recommended dosage

One of the major concerns regarding creatine use among adolescents is that teens are getting much of their information from the wrong sources, and, subsequently, are not taking creatine correctly. For instance, a recent Internet search of "creatine dosage" performed by the authors using a popular search engine resulted in more than 1 million Internet sites. In addition, there are hundreds of products on the market that contain creatine monohydrate, as well as some of the newer formulations of creatine (eg, creatine ethyl ester and magnesium-citrate chelate), each of which has its own label recommendations for dosing. With all of this information, it is surprising that there have been studies specifically designed to try and elucidate appropriate creatine dosing.

Most studies have used and tested creatine supplementation using a loading regimen, usually 20 to 30 g/d for 2 to 10 days. This regimen seems to increase stores of total creatine within the muscle by 15% to 30% [42]; however, Hultman and colleagues [40] showed that taking 3 g/d for 28 days resulted in the same increase in total muscle creatine concentration as taking 20 g/d for 6 days followed by a 2-g/d maintenance regimen. This study also showed that after the initial loading phase, muscle creatine concentration was maintained with a 2-g/d regimen. This latter fact was corroborated in other studies [42,43].

Longer-term studies of creatine use also showed that there may be a slow decrease in muscle creatine over time, despite continued supplementation [44]. This is the primary reason why "cycling" came into being. Currently, most creatine regimens recommended by manufacturers include three phases: a loading phase (1 week), a maintenance phase (5–8 weeks), and an off-cycle phase (2–4 weeks). The belief is that this type of regimen will help to counteract the slow decrease in muscle creatine over time.

There also has been some research (and even more marketing) with different forms of creatine and creatine mixtures to try to enhance its effect. Although overall results showed that there is likely little effect of any of these above the effects of creatine itself, there has been some evidence to show that ingestion of caffeine with creatine may negate its effects, whereas ingestion of large carbohydrate loads with creatine may enhance cellular uptake [36]. The load of carbohydrates required to attain this effect is large, however, and certainly health effects related to repeated large loads of carbohydrates may preclude this regimen's potential advantage.

Ergogenic value

A major controversy still exists surrounding the question of whether creatine really works as a performance-enhancing supplement. Multiple review articles in the last 10 years have come to the conclusion that creatine is effective at increasing power/force in short bouts of near maximal to maximal exertion and increasing performance with repeated efforts of maximal exertion [36,42,45,46]. In a 2005 review, Bemben and Lamont [43] looked at all of the literature on creatine as an ergogenic drug since 1999 and categorized the findings based on the type of outcomes measured. Their findings reiterated previous findings, but more specifically, showed that creatine supplementation seems to be most beneficial if dynamic or isotonic peak force is assessed as the outcome measure. Conversely, isokinetic studies have had mixed results, and measures of changes in isometric parameters showed that there is likely little benefit of creatine supplementation.

There has been significant discussion with regard to the reasons why studies involving the ergogenic value of creatine have shown mixed results. One of the most highly discussed reasons for this is the idea of "responders" versus "nonresponders." This was highlighted by Lemon [47] in 2002, who noted that some of the early studies of muscle creatine concentrations after loading showed that, although the average increase in concentration was 15% to 30%, some study participants had minimal to no increase in muscle creatine concentration. It seems that this effect is related to preloading muscle creatine concentration; participants with higher levels of creatine before supplementation seem to have less increase in muscle creatine with supplementation.

Ergogenic value in adolescents

Although creatine has been studied meticulously in adults, there is significantly less information regarding the ergogenic value of the substance in adolescents. There are studies, although rare, which showed that creatine is likely to be effective as a performance enhancer in teenagers as well. The first study of this type looked at the effect of creatine on competitive swimming. In this article, Grindstaff and colleagues [48] showed that 9 days of creatine supplementation improved the athletes' (mean age, 15.3 years) performance in a 100-m swim; however, they also showed that creatine decreased swim times in subsequent 100-m swims. A similar effect of creatine was shown later in a trial by Theodorou and colleagues [49], which was not placebo controlled, involving swimmers (mean age, 17.8 years). A later study of soccer players (mean age, 16.6 years) by Ostojic [50] showed that creatine supplementation improved soccer-specific activities, specifically sprint power, dribbling test, and vertical jump. Although this is far from conclusive evidence, these trends seem to indicate that there may be an ergogenic value of creatine in adolescents as well.

Adverse effects

At conventional doses, creatine seems to be safe in healthy athletes, although long-term data (beyond 2–3 months of use) are sparse. Numerous minor adverse effects have been reported, most of which are anecdotal in nature and not supported by scientific data. There have been several case reports of more serious adverse effects in which creatine was not clearly causative. Most controlled studies report a complete absence of side effects, do not address the issue of side effects, or report no difference in the incidence of side effects between creatine and placebo [51]; however, some of the studies investigating adverse effects have potential bias that is due to funding by supplement manufacturers [52–54]. Further limiting extrapolation of research findings to the playing field, most studies of adverse effects have tested conventional doses, and surveys have indicated that most creatine users exceed the recommended maintenance dose; therefore, the actual incidence of adverse effects may be higher than reported [1,55]. Also, most of the safety data derives from studies of athletes of collegiate age or older, although one adolescent study reported no adverse effects [50].

Weight gain is the most well-documented side effect (0.5–2 kg in the first 2 weeks); it probably is due to water retention within muscle, which may be advantageous or disadvantageous, depending on the particular sport [52,53,56–58]. In one study, after a standard 5-day creatine load, subjects gained an average of 1.04 kg, with men gaining 1.6 kg (2.0% of body weight) and women gaining 0.45 kg (0.8% of body weight) [59].

Frequently, gastrointestinal (GI) side effects are reported anecdotally, including nausea, diarrhea, dyspepsia, and abdominal pain, possibly due to malabsorption of high doses of creatine [51]; however, most studies do not indicate an increase in these symptoms compared with placebo. In one study, 3 of 87 subjects taking creatine discontinued use because of intolerable nausea (1 subject) or diarrhea (2 subjects) [60]. In a retrospective study, several subjects reported GI upset (excessive gas, diarrhea) during the loading phase [53]. The incidence of GI side effects may be lower with dissolved powder than with capsule forms of creatine [58]. Other adverse effects that have been reported include rash, dyspnea, anxiety, headache, and fatigue [56].

The greatest safety concern with creatine is renal function; a large body of research indicates that creatine supplementation has no detrimental effect on renal function in healthy athletes, including longer-term studies of up to 5.6 years [51–53,59–64]. Creatine may cause reversible elevation of serum creatinine (up to ~30%) in athletes with normal renal function [52,53,56,59,62,63,65], without causing a decrement in glomerular filtration rate as measured by creatinine clearance (which remains unchanged because urine creatinine concentration increases concomitantly) or other methods [51,61]. There are several possible explanations for this increase: (1) the increased muscle pool of creatine, which subsequently is converted to creatinine [51,65]; (2) creatine and creatinine cross-reactivity in commonly used laboratory assays [1,60]; and (3) the ability of athletes to maintain a greater training volume and intensity because of creatine's ergogenic effect, with increased creatine turnover [52,53,63]. Proteinuria has not been found to occur with creatine use [51,60,64,65]. It remains possible that high doses of creatine over long periods of time may cause renal dysfunction [1]. One must also consider that the trials investigating the renal effects of creatine were conducted primarily in healthy, active, young men. This is the patient population that is most likely to use creatine; however, it limits the ability to draw safety conclusions for other populations [61]. Data on the effects of creatine on renal function and serum creatinine concentrations in patients who have renal disease or other comorbidities are not available [61]. The slight increase in creatinine that normally is observed with creatine use may confound the estimation of renal function in athletes who have renal disease [61,65], and, as an amino acid by-product, creatine theoretically may worsen renal function in such patients [58].

Creatine has been studied and found to have no clinically significant effect on blood pressure [58,59], liver enzymes [51–53,62,63], electrolytes [52], glucose [52], uric acid [53], hematologic parameters [52,53,59,62], or muscle enzymes [52,59,62]. Some studies indicated a modest favorable effect on lipid parameters of uncertain clinical significance [52,53]. There have been anecdotal reports of muscle cramps and stiffness, musculotendinous injury, dehydration, and heat illness, but the research to date indicates that creatine does not increase the incidence of these effects [4,43,51–54]. The incidence of musculoskeletal injuries and heat illness actually may be decreased by creatine [54]; however, there is evidence that creatine may increase muscle compartmental pressures in the leg [58].

Several case reports of more serious adverse effects are found in the literature. These include:

New onset of lone atrial fibrillation during the creatine loading phase [66]

Interstitial nephritis and focal tubular injury in a previously healthy 20-year-old man taking creatine, 20 g/d, for 4 weeks, which resolved with discontinuation of creatine [67].

Worsening renal function (elevated serum creatinine and decline in glomerular filtration rate) after initiating a standard-dose regimen of creatine in a 25-year-old man who had focal segmental glomerulosclerosis and frequently relapsing steroid-responsive nephrotic syndrome, taking a therapeutic dose of cyclosporine. His renal function normalized 1 month after stopping creatine [68].

Rhabdomyolysis and acute renal failure following arthroscopic anterior cruciate ligament reconstruction in a 21-year-old, previously healthy college football player who had been taking creatine preoperatively, up to 10 g/d for 6 weeks, with full recovery [69].

Acute quadriceps compartment syndrome and rhabdomyolysis in a 24-year-old male bodybuilder taking creatine, 25 g/d, and no other supplements or anabolic steroids, after a lower extremity resistance training session. He underwent fasciotomy, had a complicated postoperative course, and at 6 months, his quadriceps strength was just 60% of his baseline strength. The investigators stated that creatine may have predisposed him to compartment syndrome by increasing water content in the muscle cells, and, thus, increasing baseline compartment pressures, a hypothesis that has some scientific support [55,58].

The Physician's Desk Reference states that contraindications to creatine use include renal failure and other renal disorders, including nephrotic syndrome, and it should be avoided in children, adolescents, pregnant women, nursing mothers, diabetics, and other persons at risk for renal disease [56]. Because of theoretic concerns of dehydration and heat illness, athletes taking creatine are recommended to drink six to eight glasses of water per day [56]. Other sources also recommend that athletes who have known or suspected renal disease or who are taking nephrotoxic medications should avoid creatine [64,65]. Because of the relative lack of long-term safety data, some investigators recommend laboratory monitoring of liver, muscle, and kidney function, including testing for proteinuria under resting conditions (after ≥20 hours of physical inactivity) [58,61].

Safety is less certain for adolescent and younger athletes, and some authorities, including the American College of Sports Medicine, conclude that physicians should recommend against creatine use in adolescents

[1,56,57]. Also, its effects on other creatine-containing tissues, such as the brain, cardiac muscle, and testes, are unknown [4]. There also is concern that creatine may function as a "gateway substance" that may prompt a young athlete to consider other ergogenic aids, such as anabolic steroids [1]. Overall, however, the published literature provides an excellent safety record for creatine supplementation at standard dosages, with the foregoing caveats kept in mind.

Beta-hydroxy-beta-methylbutyrate

HMB, a metabolite of the essential branched-chain amino acid (BCAA) leucine, is produced endogenously in small amounts and contained in foods such as catfish, citrus fruits, and breast milk [22]. It also is known as hydroxymethylbutyrate, beta-hydroxyisovalerate, and 3-hydroxyisovalerate [70]. It is promoted as an "anticatabolic" agent that exerts an anabolic effect by suppressing protein breakdown and cellular damage after intense exercise, thereby allowing quicker recovery and increased lean body mass and strength [4,46,57]. HMB also is a cholesterol precursor, and its promotion of muscle growth may be due to its provision of a larger supply of cholesterol for cell membrane synthesis to "patch up" local deficiencies of membrane cholesterol that are believed to occur with muscular hypertrophy [71]. It also may have immunomodulatory properties [70]. HMB may be attractive to adolescents because of its purported "muscle-building" effects that may positively affect physical appearance, regardless of its effect on muscle performance [72].

The typical dosage of HMB is 1.5 to 3 g/d. Higher dosages do not seem to offer additional benefit [71,73,74]. Most of the studies investigating the effect of HMB on muscle strength and body composition have been 3 to 8 weeks in duration. In one of the original studies of HMB, a dosage of 1.5 to 3 g/d improved strength and muscle mass gains in untrained subjects undertaking a resistance-training regimen [75]. Other studies have corroborated these findings [4,46,57,71,74]; however, studies have found little to no benefit for trained athletes [4,46,76]. This may be explained by the fact that physical training itself stimulates adaptation in the athlete, such that subsequent exercise is accompanied by less protein turnover and breakdown (ie, training has an anticatabolic effect). Therefore, trained athletes would receive less, if any, benefit from an anticatabolic agent like HMB [74]. From a muscle damage standpoint, HMB was shown to reduce levels of markers of muscle damage (eg, creatine phosphokinase, lactate dehydrogenase) after exercise, such as distance running and weight training [75,77]. These outcomes, however, are merely surrogate end points for the athlete who seeks to realize accelerated recovery from exercise sessions, and studies examining the effect of HMB on real-life outcomes, such as delayed-onset muscle soreness, have been conflicting [78,79]. One interpretation of the available evidence is that although it seems that HMB may enhance the untrained athlete's initial adaptation to resistance training in the short-term (3–8 weeks), nonusers eventually will "catch up," such that HMB probably does not enhance the athlete's ultimate performance potential that is achieved by optimal training without supplementation. Although HMB has not been studied in this manner, it may be useful for a 4- to 8-week period at the beginning of training, after which it may be discontinued without detrimental effect.

There are no reported adverse effects of HMB in limited short-term studies, including no changes in blood pressure, liver enzymes, lipid profile, renal function, electrolytes (except a decrease in bicarbonate level of unclear significance), hematologic parameters, urinalysis, testosterone, cortisol, or male fertility [4,70,80,81]. There are no contraindications, although the Physician's Desk References advises to avoid HMB in pregnant and lactating women [70]. No studies exist in adolescents or in long-term supplementation, and one investigator advises physicians to recommend against use by adolescent athletes until more data are accumulated [67].

Protein and amino acids

Athletes use protein supplements to increase body mass and strength and enhance recovery from exercise. Although athletes, especially strength-trained athletes, are known to require more dietary protein than nonathletes to maintain a positive nitrogen balance, intake of excess protein does not provide additional gains in strength or mass [82]. Although the recommended protein intake for sedentary individuals is 0.8 to 1.0 g/kg/d, strength-trained athletes require 1.6 to 1.7 g/kg/d, which is not difficult to achieve from whole food sources [46,82]. There is no evidence that ingesting protein above recommended levels improves muscle growth; however, protein supplements may be useful to meet bodily needs for athletes who ingest inadequate amounts in their diets (eg, vegetarians, athletes following restrictive diets) [46].

There is evidence, however, that the timing and composition of protein/amino acid intake in relation to exercise sessions may affect the athlete's physiologic response to training. For optimal muscle anabolism following exercise, amino acids must be made available to the muscle, and adequate insulin must be present to enable muscle to use them. It is known that certain amino acids stimulate insulin release. Postexercise ingestion of a "recovery drink" containing insulinotropic amino acids with carbohydrate stimulates increased pancreatic insulin release, which stimulates muscle anabolism. Of these amino acids, leucine seems to be most important. A protein supplement that contains amino acids in dipeptide and tripeptide forms results in the most rapid increase in blood amino acid levels following exercise, because these forms are absorbed fastest by the GI tract. Protein hydrolysates, such as whey protein and casein protein, contain amino acids in these forms and may be advantageous to the strength-trained athlete [83].

There are several particular amino acids that are used by athletes and merit discussion. Glutamine is known to be used by immune cells, and some athletes use protein hydrolysate supplements enriched with glutamine in an attempt to optimize immune function along with the previously mentioned anabolic effects [46,82,83]. The BCAAs leucine, isoleucine, and valine are purported to aid in endurance exercise by counteracting central fatigue, possibly by interfering with tryptophan kinetics or other mechanisms [72,84–87]. Supplements containing BCAAs may prove to be helpful for sports such as tennis, soccer, distance running, cycling, and swimming [72]. The research has been conflicting, and further study is needed [84,85]. One recent study of elite outrigger canoeists found that 6 weeks of leucine supplementation (45 mg/kg/d) significantly increased time to exhaustion and peak upper body power and decreased the rating of perceived exertion throughout a 55-minute period of rowing [88]. The investigators noted that most previous studies of leucine in exercise used single or multiple doses on the day of testing, whereas their study used leucine for a 6-week period before testing [88]. The catabolism of BCAAs is thiamine dependent, and the use of them may require increased thiamine intake [72]. Several other amino acids are known to stimulate growth hormone secretion (arginine, lysine, and ornithine) and increase nitric oxide synthesis (arginine) in addition to their direct role in protein synthesis [46,86]. Whether they have any ergogenic effect, however, is unclear [86]. It remains possible that there exists optimal combinations of amino acids, including those described above, that will produce significant ergogenic effects, and the concoction may vary for different athletic activities.

Stimulants

Caffeine

Caffeine, a trimethylxanthine with stimulant properties, has strong evidence of ergogenicity. Approximately 27% of adolescent athletes in the United States report caffeine use for performance enhancement [89]. In athletics, it is used mainly for enhancement of submaximal aerobic and endurance activities [46,89]. It may have other applications, such as team sports. Caffeine has a myriad of physiologic effects, on the central nervous system and on peripheral body systems, which contribute to its ergogenic effects. Caffeine's key physiologic mechanism may be adenosine receptor antagonism [90]. Adenosine inhibits central nervous system (CNS) neurotransmission, decreases catecholamine release, and inhibits lipolysis; caffeine affects all of these in the opposite manner (CNS stimulation, increased catecholamine release and lipolysis) [46,72,90]. Regular caffeine use causes up-regulation of adenosine receptors, which may contribute to tolerance in habitual users [90]. CNS activity may be affected by caffeine through other mechanisms as well [57,82]. Stimulation of lipolysis functions to mobilize free fatty acids to be used by exercising muscle, thus sparing glycogen stores [72]. Other mechanisms may include increased contractility of skeletal and cardiac muscle (by way of mobilization of intracellular calcium, sensitization of myofibrils to calcium, and other mechanisms) [57,72,82], increased metabolic rate [23], increased cortisol levels [46], and antioxidant activity [46]. Caffeine is known to increase heart rate and blood pressure [46]. It is absorbed rapidly from the GI tract, with 90% cleared from the stomach within 20 minutes of ingestion, peak plasma concentrations reached in 40 to 60 minutes, and a half-life of 3 to 5 hours [90].

Caffeine may produce ergogenic effects at doses as low as 250 mg (3.0–3.5 mg/kg body weight) [82]; most studies showing benefit used doses around 400 to 600 mg [90], and on a body-weight basis, a reasonable dose would be 5 mg/kg [72]. In the past, caffeine was banned by the World Anti-Doping Agency (WADA) above a threshold urinary concentration, but in 2007 it is legal at any level [91]; however, the NCAA has set an upper legal limit of 15 μg/mL in urine [92]. A 100-mg dose of caffeine increases urine levels by approximately 1.5 μg/mL; therefore, 800 to 1000 mg would need to be ingested to approach the legal limit [90]. Because exercise reduces the urinary excretion of caffeine, however, the correlation between oral dose and subsequent urine concentration is unpredictable [72]. Most studies have used caffeine in capsule form. In comparison with caffeine ingested in coffee, plasma caffeine levels are similar, but enhancement of endurance is observed only when caffeine is consumed independent of coffee, indicating that there are substances in coffee that antagonize the ergogenic effects of caffeine [90]. Caffeine also may be effective in "defizzed" soft drinks, which also provide a source of simple carbohydrate, although the caffeine concentration is low in this form. This practice is common among endurance and ultradistance athletes [90]. Caffeine's positive effect occurs regardless of whether it is ingested in single or multiple doses or before or during exercise, and its effect seems to be prolonged as much as 6 hours postingestion [90]; however, its benefits may depend on abstinence for several days before use [72], and its effect is more pronounced in relative nonusers (<50 mg/d) than in regular users (>300 mg/d) [90].

Caffeine was shown to reduce perception of fatigue and increase time to exhaustion in submaximal exercise of 30- to 60-minute duration (running and cycling) [46,89]. It also was shown to reduce times to run a set distance and to improve 1500-m swim times [90]. Caffeine does not seem to be useful for sprinting or short-burst activity [46,72], but it may be effective for sports involving repeated short bursts of activity interspersed in more prolonged activity, as in tennis and team sports [90,93]. During periods of sleep deprivation, caffeine improves alertness, neurocognitive performance, and aerobic performance [23,90].

Common adverse effects of caffeine are insomnia, tremors, headache [23], anxiety [57], flushing [72], palpitations [46], premature ventricular contractions [90], and supraventricular arrhythmias [23]. Caffeine is believed to have a diuretic effect, but it seems not to have this effect when used immediately before exercise, and there is no evidence that it causes dehydration

[57,72]. Habitual caffeine use produces physiologic dependence, in which the body's "normal" state becomes the caffeinated state, and performance declines in its absence [23]. Withdrawal symptoms, including headache, irritability, decreased alertness, difficulty concentrating, and increased fatigue, occur as soon as 12 hours after cessation of use in habituated users [90]. There is concern that caffeine may increase core body temperature [90]. Of greatest concern are the reports of sudden deaths in athletes taking supplements containing caffeine and ephedra. None of these events occurred with supplements containing only caffeine, however, and the deaths were believed to be due to ephedra [90]. As with most dietary supplements, there is much more scientific evidence in adult subjects than in adolescents, and although adult studies indicate safety of use, some investigators contend that there is not enough evidence to make recommendations regarding the use and safety of caffeine in adolescents [57].

Ephedra and other stimulants

Ephedra sinica, also known as Chinese ephedra or ma huang, is a shrub native to northern China and Mongolia. It contains ephedrine alkaloids, including ephedrine (the primary alkaloid), pseudoephedrine, norephedrine, and norpseudoephedrine, that mediate its physiologic effects. There is an ephedra species native to North America, *Ephedra americana*, which has no ephedrine alkaloid content [94]. Ephedrine has been used traditionally as a cold remedy. Other sports-related uses include weight loss, appetite suppression, increased alertness, and improved performance when fatigued [2,4,23,57]. There is little evidence of any benefit to ephedra use for athletic purposes [94]. Ephedra was banned by the FDA in 2004 because of numerous severe adverse effects associated with it, including several deaths, and it is banned by virtually all amateur and professional sports-governing bodies [94]. It is a sympathomimetic, with CNS, cardiovascular, and metabolic effects mediated directly and indirectly by way of catecholamine release [94,95]. It has a myriad of adverse effects, including hypertension, insomnia, anxiety, tremors, headache, dependence, psychosis, nephrolithiasis, seizures, arrhythmias, strokes, myocardial infarction, and several deaths [23,57,94,96]. It may still be available to athletes by way of the Internet. Ephedra's risks clearly outweigh its benefits; it is obvious that the physician's recommendation must be that ephedra should not be used by any athlete for any purpose.

Since ephedra was banned, many supplement manufacturers have replaced it with *Citrus aurantium*. Other names for this botanical are bitter orange, Seville orange, sour orange, Zhi shi (Chinese), Kijitsu (Japanese), and Chisil (Korean) [97]. It contains synephrine, also a sympathomimetic, which has similar effects as other ephedrine alkaloids, although it is a milder stimulant than ephedrine [23]. *Citrus aurantium* is banned by the NCAA but not by the WADA [91,92]. It has been studied for weight loss only in combination with other substances (caffeine, ephedrine, and others), and even then there is no long-term evidence of efficacy [98]. Elevated blood pressure has been observed with *Citrus aurantium*, and drug interactions are likely because it is a potent inhibitor of the cytochrome p450 enzyme CYP3A4 [97]. There have been case reports of myocardial infarction, variant angina, ischemic colitis, seizure, syncope, and stroke associated with its use [98–101]. Athletes should be strongly advised to avoid these supplements as well.

Alkalotic agents

The most commonly used agents in this class are sodium bicarbonate ($NaHCO_3$) and sodium citrate. They are used to delay fatigue and improve high-intensity anaerobic exercise performance [46]. They are believed to work by increasing extracellular pH, thus enhancing the extracellular buffer capacity. During high-intensity exercise, glycolysis produces lactic acid, which dissociates into hydrogen ions (H^+) and lactate, which decrease intracellular pH. At lower intracellular pH, glycolytic enzyme activity is inhibited and fatigue ensues. By increasing the extracellular pH and increasing the pH gradient across the cell membrane, alkalotic agents delay the decrease in intracellular pH by enhancing efflux of H^+ and lactate out of the myocyte, hence improving contractile activity and delaying fatigue [102]. Their effect on performance may involve other mechanisms, including CNS effects and increased plasma volume [103].

Study results, however, have been conflicting. They may be beneficial only for exercise activities in which the acidosis of exercise is the limiting factor in performance. If the exercise task does not use fully the body's endogenous buffer system, then augmenting with buffering agents would not be expected to improve performance. This may be why studies generally have not shown alkalotic agents to be beneficial for exercise lasting less than 30 seconds or in strength/resistance exercise [46,102]. Studies failing to show benefit may be limited by insufficient dosing, the exercise protocol itself (failure to challenge the body's buffering capacity), characteristics of study subjects (eg, elite, anaerobically trained athletes familiar with the exercise protocol may benefit more than less-trained subjects), or other factors [102,104]. High-intensity exercise (80%–125% of Vo_2 max for 1–7 minutes) that involves large muscle groups and recruits fast motor units is most likely to benefit (eg, mountain bike downhills, track and road cycling, running [800–3000 m distance, possibly up to 10,000 m], and prolonged intermittent bouts of intense exercise as in team sports) [46,102,105,106]. Although alkalotic agents do not increase time to exhaustion, they have been shown to decrease rating of perceived exertion at a given intensity and improve 5000-m running time by 30 seconds in trained collegiate runners [103].

Alkalotic agents are legal in all jurisdictions but may cause a problem for athletes undergoing drug testing. Because they cause urine alkalinization, which can mask the presence of some banned substances, the athlete may be withheld at the point of testing until urine pH normalizes [102]. For sodium bicarbonate, 0.3 g/kg body weight seems to be the minimally effective dose, and it is unclear whether higher doses provide greater benefit. The increase in pH peaks at 100 to 120 minutes postingestion. For sodium citrate, 0.5 g/kg is the most effective dose, and pH peaks at 120 minutes postingestion [102]. Sodium bicarbonate also has been studied in a chronic dosing regimen (0.3–0.5 g/kg daily for 5–6 days) and was shown to improve performance similarly to acute dosing, with the alkalotic effect persisting for up to 2 days after the final dose [104]. Both agents are limited by GI side effects (nausea, cramps, diarrhea), which may be problematic during the 60 to 120 minutes before exercise [103,104]. Chronic daily dosing offers the potential advantage of circumventing these side effects [104]. Excessive doses of alkalotic agents are known to cause severe metabolic alkalosis (with complications such as arrhythmias and respiratory failure), and there have been several reports of gastric rupture due to bicarbonate conversion to carbon dioxide in the stomach, although none of these is known to have occurred in athletic situations [107].

Glycerol

Glycerol is an osmotically active molecule that is used to optimize hydration status for the purpose of improving performance in warm conditions [108]. It acutely (up to 4 hours) increases total body water, but as a prehydration method it has had conflicting results in studies of exercise performance [108,109]. Also, when used for "hyperhydration" before exercise, it has had adverse effects of GI upset, headache, and blurred vision [109]; however, a recent study showed that rehydration with glycerol after an exercise session inducing dehydration (4% body weight) significantly improved time to exhaustion in a subsequent exercise session 90 minutes later in trained male cyclists, compared with rehydration with water alone. None of the subjects experienced adverse effects [109]. Glycerol has been shown to be safe in doses of up to 5 g/kg body weight [109]. It may be useful for athletes who undertake multiple exercise sessions daily (eg, football players in preseason practices, all-day tournaments in other team and individual sports).

Vitamins and minerals

The dietary reference intakes for all known vitamins and essential minerals are available at http://www.iom.edu/Object.File/Master/21/372/0.pdf. As a general rule, there is no benefit to supplementation of vitamins and minerals above the recommended daily amounts. With an adequately balanced diet, the athlete without any medical condition that predisposes to vitamin deficiency will not enhance performance by supplemental intake [46]; however, athletes who follow restrictive diets may benefit from supplementation if their diet does not provide recommended amounts [23]. It may be reasonable to recommend that athletes who are at risk for, or concerned about, micronutrient deficiency take a daily multivitamin supplement. Several micronutrients are discussed further.

Iron supplements are used commonly by athletes for performance enhancement, a practice that can be helpful or harmful. In the presence of iron-deficiency anemia, which is more common in young athletes than in the general population, supplementation is clearly beneficial for performance [46,110]; however, the diagnosis can be difficult to establish in athletes. In response to training, hemoglobin concentration decreases transiently as the plasma volume expands to a greater degree than does red cell mass, the so-called "sports anemia." Ferritin levels also decrease, but this usually does not indicate true iron deficiency. An elevated serum transferrin receptor level is a more specific indicator of iron deficiency than is a low ferritin level in athletes, rendering it a useful test in this case. Studies of iron supplementation showed objective performance improvement only in athletes who had iron-deficiency anemia or untrained individuals with low ferritin levels. Athletes with normal or low ferritin levels do not benefit from supplementation. The risks for empiric iron supplementation include overlooking a serious medical condition that presents with anemia (eg, celiac disease, occult gastrointestinal bleeding, gynecologic disease), as well as the complications of iron overload, including hemochromatosis and diabetes mellitus [110].

Chromium is an essential trace element that is used by athletes for modifying body composition (eg, muscle building, decreasing body fat). It is most commonly ingested as chromium picolinate in quantities that provide approximately 100 times the recommended amount because of greater bioavailability compared with dietary chromium; however, a large body of scientific evidence indicates that chromium has no effect on body composition when taken in this form, and there are serious concerns for the potential adverse effects of chromium accumulation within the body. Evidence of mutagenicity has been found in animal studies, and there have been human reports of anemia, thrombocytopenia, hepatic dysfunction, renal failure, rhabdomyolysis, dermatitis, neurologic disturbances, hypoglycemia, and exanthematous pustulosis [111].

The Gateway Theory

In addition to their inherent risks, the adolescent use of dietary supplements has been linked to an increased risk for using illegal performance-enhancing substances (eg, anabolic steroids, growth hormone, erythropoietin) [3]. Dodge and Jaccard [34], in their analysis of the Add Health database

(~ 15,000 respondents), found that adolescents who report the use of any legal ergogenic supplement are nearly 26 times more likely to report the use of anabolic steroids compared with adolescents who do not report the use of legal supplements. This relationship is concerning, because it indicates that the use of legal dietary supplements may function as a "stepping stone" or "gateway" to illegal or more harmful types of substance use. Although this relationship has been observed in other types of substance abuse, such as alcohol, tobacco, and marijuana, the potential for dietary supplements to function similarly remains to be clarified [3].

The Gateway Theory is complex and involves three interrelated hypotheses. "Sequencing" implies that there is a fixed relationship between two substances, such that one substance is regularly initiated before the other. "Association" implies that initiation of one substance increases the likelihood of initiation of the second substance. "Causation" implies that the use of the first substance actually causes the use of the second substance [112]. The Gateway Theory predicts a positive, sequential relationship between the use of legal substances (eg, ergogenic dietary supplements) and the use of illicit substances (eg, anabolic steroids), in which the use of legal substances is followed by the use of illegal substances [34]. This relationship may be causative, such that the use of legal substances causes a person to proceed to using illicit substances, although such a relationship has never been proven. Alternatively, it is possible that the use of ergogenic supplements and anabolic steroids is part of a "problem behavior cluster," a hypothesis that risky behaviors in adolescents often co-occur because adolescents learn risk behaviors together, learn it is socially appropriate to engage in such behaviors simultaneously, or the behaviors share some other underlying cause. Dodge and Jaccard [34] found a low correlation between performance-enhancing substance use and other "risky" behaviors, such as binge drinking, drug use, and injectable drug use; hence they concluded that their findings are better explained by the Gateway Theory.

Regardless of whether the relationship between legal supplement use and anabolic steroid use is causative, or merely sequential or associational, there is practical application to adolescent medical care. At preparticipation examinations and routine health maintenance visits, the physician should inquire about past and present ergogenic dietary supplement use and whether the patient is considering using supplements in the future. This will identify patients who may benefit from education about legal supplements and more extensive counseling about the risks and consequences of illegal performance-enhancing substance use.

References

[1] Laos C, Metzl JD. Performance-enhancing drug use in young athletes. Adolesc Med 2006; 17:719–31.

[2] The National Collegiate Athletic Association. NCAA study of substance use of college student-athletes. Available at: http://www.ncaa.org/library/research/substance_use_habits/2006/2006_substance_use_report.pdf. Accessed December 28, 2006.

[3] Dorsch KD, Bell A. Dietary supplement use in adolescents. Curr Opin Pediatr 2005;17(5): 653–7.

[4] Tokish JM, Kocher MS, Hawkins RJ. Ergogenic aids: a review of basic science, performance, side effects, and status in sports. Am J Sports Med 2004;32(6):1543–53.

[5] Wollschlaeger B. The dietary supplement and health education act and supplements: dietary and nutritional supplements need no more regulations. Int J Toxicol 2003;22(5): 387–90.

[6] Center for Food Safety and Applied Nutrition, U.S. Food and Drug Administration. Dietary supplement health and education act of 1994. Available at: http://www.cfsan.fda.gov/~;dms/dietsupp.html. Accessed November 12, 2006.

[7] Siegner AW. The food and drug administration's actions on ephedra and androstenedione: understanding their potential impacts on the protections of the dietary supplement health and education act. Food Drug Law J 2004;59(4):617–28.

[8] Turner RE, Degnan FH, Archer DL. Label claims for foods and supplements: a review of the regulations. Nutr Clin Pract 2005;20(1):21–32.

[9] Hathcock J. Dietary supplements: how they are used and regulated. J Nutr 2001;131: 1114S–7S.

[10] Center for Food Safety and Applied Nutrition, U.S. Food and Drug Administration. Overview of dietary supplements. Available at: http://www.cfsan.fda.gov/~;dms/ds-oview.html. Accessed November 12, 2006.

[11] Center for Food Safety and Applied Nutrition, Office of Nutritional Products, Labeling, and Dietary Supplements, U.S. Food and Drug Administration. New dietary ingredients in dietary supplements. Available at: http://www.cfsan.fda.gov/~;dms/ds3strfs.html. Accessed December 3, 2006.

[12] Noonan C, Noonan WP. Marketing dietary supplements in the United States: a review of the requirements for new dietary ingredients. Toxicology 2006;221(1):4–8.

[13] Larsen LL, Berry JA. The regulation of dietary supplements. J Am Acad Nurse Pract 2003; 15(9):410–4.

[14] Center for Food Safety and Applied Nutrition, U.S. Food and Drug Administration. Claims that can be made for conventional foods and dietary supplements. Available at: http://www.cfsan.fda.gov/~;dms/hclaims.html. Accessed December 3, 2006.

[15] Center for Food Safety and Applied Nutrition, Office of Nutritional Products, Labeling, and Dietary Supplements, U.S. Food and Drug Administration. Fact sheet on FDA's strategy for dietary supplements. Available at: http://www.cfsan.fda.gov/~;dms/ds3strfs.html. Accessed November 12, 2006.

[16] Bonakdar RA. Integrative medicine: herb-drug interactions: what physicians need to know. Available at: http://www.patientcareonline.com/patcare/article/articleDetail.jsp?id=111668&;SearchString=bonakdar. Accessed January 6, 2007.

[17] Catlin DH, Leder BZ, Ahrens B, et al. Trace contamination of over-the-counter androstenedione and positive urine test results for a nandrolone metabolite. JAMA 2000;284: 2618–21.

[18] Baume N, Mahler N, Kamber M, et al. Research of stimulants and anabolic steroids in dietary supplements. Scand J Med Sci Sports 2006;16(1):41–8.

[19] Green GA, Catlin DH, Starcevic B. Analysis of over-the-counter dietary supplements. Clin J Sport Med 2001;11(4):254–9.

[20] Maughan RJ. Contamination of dietary supplements and positive drug tests in sport. J Sports Sci 2005;23(9):883–9.

[21] Striegel H, Vollkommer G, Horstmann T, et al. Contaminated nutritional supplements—legal protection for elite athletes who tested positive: a case report from Germany. J Sports Sci 2005;23(7):723–6.

[22] Armsey TD, Hosey RG. Medical aspects of sports: epidemiology of injuries, preparticipation physical examination, and drugs in sports. Clin Sports Med 2004;23(2):255–79.

[23] Lombardo JA. Supplements and athletes. South Med J 2004;97(9):877–9.

[24] ConsumerLab.com. Available at: http://www.consumerlab.com. Accessed February 3, 2007.

[25] National Sanitation Foundation (NSF) International. Available at: http://www.nsf.org. Accessed February 3, 2007.

[26] U.S. Pharmacopeia's Dietary Supplement Verification Program. Available at: http://www.usp.org. Accessed February 3, 2007.

[27] The National Collegiate Athletic Association. NCAA study of substance use and abuse habits of college student-athletes. Available at: http://www.ncaa.org/sports_sciences/education/199709abuse.pdf. Accessed January 7, 2007.

[28] Smith J, Dahm D. Creatine use among a select population of high school athletes. Mayo Clin Proc 2000;75:1257–63.

[29] Ray T, Eck J, Convington R, et al. Use of oral creatine as an ergogenic aid for increased sports performance: perceptions of adolescent athletes. South Med J 2001;94(6):608–12.

[30] Metzl J, Small E, Levine S, et al. Creatine use among young athletes. Pediatrics 2001;108: 421–5.

[31] Mcguine TA, Sullivan JC, Berhardt DT. Creatine supplementation in high school football players. Clin J Sport Med 2001;11:247–53.

[32] Bell A, Dorsch K, McCreary D, et al. A look at nutritional supplement use in adolescents. J Adolesc Health 2004;34:508–16.

[33] Wilson K, Klein J, Sesselberg T, et al. Use of complimentary medicine and dietary supplements among U.S. adolescents. J Adolesc Health 2006;38:385–94.

[34] Dodge TL, Jaccard JJ. The effect of high school sports participation on the use of performance-enhancing substances in young adulthood. J Adolesc Health 2006;39:367–73.

[35] Bloch K, Schoenheimer R. The biological precursors of creatine. J Biolumin Chemilumin 1941;138:167–94.

[36] Terjung R, Clarkson P, Eichner R, et al. The American College of Sports Medicine roundtable on the physiological and health effects of oral creatine supplementation. Med Sci Sports Exerc 2000;32(3):706–17.

[37] Wallimann T, Wyss M, Brdiczka D, et al. Intracellular compartmentation, structure and function of creatine kinase isoenzymes in tissues with high and fluctuating energy demands: the 'phosphocreatine circuit' for cellular energy homeostasis. Biochem J 1992; 281:21–40.

[38] Mommaerts W, Wallner A. The breakdown of adenosine triphosphate in the contraction cycle of the frog sartorius muscle. J Phys 1967;193:343–57.

[39] Iyengar MR. Creatine kinase as an intracellular regulator. J Muscle Res Cell Motil 1984;5: 527–34.

[40] Hultman D, Soderlund K, Timmons JA, et al. Muscle creatine loading in men. J Appl Physiol 1996;81:232–7.

[41] Haussinger D, Roth E, Lang F, et al. Cellular hydration state: an important determination of protein catabolism in health and disease. Lancet 1993;341:1330–2.

[42] Kreider R. Creatine supplementation: analysis of ergogenic value, medical safety, and concerns. Journal of Exercise Physiology Online 1998;1(1). Available at: http://faculty.css.edu/tboone2/asep/jan3.htm. Accessed January 13, 2007.

[43] Bemben MG, Lamont HS. Creatine supplementation and exercise performance: recent findings. Sports Med 2005;35(2):107–25.

[44] Derave W, Eijinde BO, Hespel P. Creatine supplementation in health and disease: what is the evidence for long term efficacy? Mol Cell Biochem 2003;244:49–55.

[45] Hespel P, Maughan RJ, Greenhaff PL. Dietary supplements for football. J Sports Sci 2006; 24(7):749–61.

[46] Ciocca M. Medication and supplement use by athletes. Clin Sports Med 2005;24:719–38.

[47] Lemon PW. Dietary creatine supplementation and exercise performance: why inconsistent results? Can J Appl Physiol 2002;27(6):663–80.

[48] Grindstaff PD, Kreider R, Bishop R, et al. Effects of creatine supplementation on repetitive sprint performance and body composition in competitive swimmers. Int J Sport Nutr 1997; 7:330–46.

[49] Theodorou AS, Havenetidis K, Zanker CL. Effects of acute creatine loading with or without carbohydrate on repeated bouts of maximal swimming in high-performance swimmers. J Strength Cond Res 2005;19(2):265–9.

[50] Ostojic SM. Creatine supplementation in young soccer players. Int J Sport Nutr Exerc Metab 2004;14:95–103.

[51] Shao A, Hathcock JN. Risk assessment for creatine monohydrate. Regul Toxicol Pharmacol 2006;45(3):242–51.

[52] Kreider RB, Melton C, Rasmussen CJ, et al. Long-term creatine supplementation does not significantly affect clinical markers of health in athletes. Mol Cell Biochem 2003;244(1–2):95–104.

[53] Schilling BK, Stone MH, Utter A, et al. Creatine supplementation and health variables: a retrospective study. Med Sci Sports Exerc 2001;33(2):183–8.

[54] Greenwood M, Kreider RB, Melton C, et al. Creatine supplementation during college football training does not increase the incidence of cramping or injury. Mol Cell Biochem 2003; 244(1–2):83–8.

[55] Robinson SJ. Acute quadriceps compartment syndrome and rhabdomyolysis in a weight lifter using high-dose creatine supplementation. J Am Board Fam Pract 2000;13(2):134–7.

[56] PDR Health. Creatine. Available at: http://www.pdrhealth.com/drug_info/nmdrugprofiles/ nutsupdrugs/cre_0086.shtml. Accessed December 30, 2006.

[57] DesJardins M. Supplement use in the adolescent athlete. Curr Sports Med Rep 2002;1: 369–73.

[58] Bizzarini E, De Angelis L. Is the use of oral creatine supplementation safe? J Sports Med Phys Fitness 2004;44(4):411–6.

[59] Mihic S, MacDonald JR, McKenzie S, et al. Acute creatine loading increases fat-free mass, but does not affect blood pressure, plasma creatinine, or CK activity in men and women. Med Sci Sports Exerc 2000;32(2):291–6.

[60] Groeneveld GJ, Beijer C, Veldink JH, et al. Few adverse effects of long-term creatine supplementation in a placebo-controlled trial. Int J Sports Med 2005;26(4):307–13.

[61] Pline KA, Smith CL. The effect of creatine intake on renal function. Ann Pharmacother 2005;39(6):1093–6.

[62] Robinson TM, Sewell DA, Casey A, et al. Dietary creatine supplementation does not affect some haematological indices, or indices of muscle damage and hepatic and renal function. Br J Sports Med 2000;34:284–8.

[63] Mayhew DL, Mayhew JL, Ware JS. Effects of long-term creatine supplementation on liver and kidney functions in American college football players. Int J Sport Nutr Exerc Metab 2002;12(4):453–60.

[64] Poortmans JR, Francaux M. Long-term oral creatine supplementation does not impair renal function in healthy athletes. Med Sci Sports Exerc 1999;31(8):1108–10.

[65] Yoshizumi WM, Tsourounis C. Effects of creatine supplementation on renal function. J Herb Pharmacother 2004;4(1):1–7.

[66] Kammer RT. Lone atrial fibrillation associated with creatine monohydrate supplementation. Pharmacotherapy 2005;25(5):762–4.

[67] Koshy KM, Griswold E, Schneeberger EE. Interstitial nephritis in a patient taking creatine. N Engl J Med 1999;340(10):814–5.

[68] Pritchard NR, Kalra PA. Renal dysfunction accompanying oral creatine supplements. Lancet 1998;351(9111):1252–3.

[69] Sheth NP, Sennett B, Berns JS. Rhabdomyolysis and acute renal failure following arthroscopic knee surgery in a college football player taking creatine supplements. Clin Nephrol 2006;65(2):134–7.

[70] PDR Health. Beta-hydroxy-beta-methylbutyrate (HMB). www.pdrhealth.com/drug_info/nmdrugprofiles/nutsupdrugs/bet_0138.shtml. Accessed December 30, 2006.

[71] Palisin T, Stacy JJ. Beta-hydroxy-beta-methylbutyrate and its use in athletics. Curr Sports Med Rep 2005;4(4):220–3.

[72] Schwenk TL, Costley CD. When food becomes a drug: nonanabolic nutritional supplement use in athletes. Am J Sports Med 2002;30(6):907–16.

[73] Gallagher PM, Carrithers JA, Godard MP, et al. β-hydroxy-β-methylbutyrate ingestion, part I: effects on strength and fat free mass. Med Sci Sports Exerc 2000;32(12): 2109–15.

[74] Slater GJ, Jenkins D. Beta-hydroxy-beta-methylbutyrate supplementation and the promotion of muscle growth and strength. Sports Med 2000;30(2):105–16.

[75] Nissen S, Sharp R, Ray M, et al. Effect of leucine metabolite beta-hydroxy-beta-methylbutyrate on muscle metabolism during resistance-exercise training. J Appl Physiol 1994;81(5): 2095–104.

[76] Slater G, Jenkins D, Logan P, et al. Beta-hydroxy-beta-methylbutyrate (HMB) supplementation does not affect changes in strength or body composition during resistance training in trained men. Int J Sport Exerc Metab 2001;11:384–96.

[77] Knitter AE, Panton L, Rathmacher JA, et al. Effects of beta-hydroxy-beta-methylbutyrate on muscle damage after a prolonged run. J Appl Physiol 2000;89:1340–4.

[78] van Someren KA, Edwards AJ, Howatson G. Supplementation with beta-hydroxy-beta-methylbutyrate (HMB) and alpha-keto-isocaproic acid (KIC) reduces signs and symptoms of exercise-induced muscle damage in man. Int J Sport Nutr Exerc Metab 2005;15(4): 413–24.

[79] Paddon-Jones D, Keech A, Jenkins D. Short-term beta-hydroxy-beta-methylbutyrate supplementation does not reduce symptoms of eccentric muscle damage. Int J Sport Nutr Exerc Metab 2001;11(4):442–50.

[80] Gallagher PM, Carrithers JA, Godard MP, et al. Beta-hydroxy-beta-methylbutyrate ingestion, part II: effects on hematology, hepatic and renal function. Med Sci Sports Exerc 2000; 32(12):2116–9.

[81] Crowe MJ, O'Connor DM, Lukins JE. The effects of beta-hydroxy-beta-methylbutyrate (HMB) and HMB/creatine supplementation on indices of health in highly trained athletes. Int J Sport Exerc Metab 2003;13(2):184–97.

[82] Ahrendt DM. Ergogenic aids: counseling the athlete. Am Fam Physician 2001;63: 913–22.

[83] Manninen AH. Hyperinsulinaemia, hyperaminoacidaemia and post-exercise muscle anabolism: the search for the optimal recovery drink. Br J Sports Med 2006;40:900–5.

[84] Newsholme EA, Blomstrand E. Branched-chain amino acids and central fatigue. J Nutr 2006;136:274S–6S.

[85] Blomstrand E. A role for branched-chain amino acids in reducing central fatigue. J Nutr 2006;136:544S–7S.

[86] Paddon-Jones D, Borsheim E, Wolfe RR. Potential ergogenic effects of arginine and creatine supplementation. J Nutr 2004;134:2888S–94S.

[87] Ohtani M, Sugita M, Maruyama K. Amino acid mixture improves training efficiency in athletes. J Nutr 2006;136:538S–43S.

[88] Crowe MJ, Weatherson JN, Bowden BF. Effects of dietary leucine supplementation on exercise performance. Eur J Appl Physiol 2006;97:664–72.

[89] Magkos F, Kavouras SA. Caffeine and ephedrine: physiological, metabolic and performance-enhancing effects. Sports Med 2004;34(13):871–89.

[90] Keisler BD, Armsey TD. Caffeine as an ergogenic aid. Curr Sports Med Rep 2006;5(4): 215–9.

[91] World Anti-Doping Agency. The 2007 prohibited list: international standard. Available at: http://www.wada-ama.org/rtecontent/document/2007_List_En.pdf. Accessed January 14, 2007.

[92] The National Collegiate Athletic Association. NCAA banned-drug classes 2006–2007. Available at: http://www1.ncaa.org/membership/ed_outreach/health-safety/drug_testing/banned_drug_classes.pdf. Accessed January 14, 2007.

[93] Stuart GR, Hopkins WG, Cook C, et al. Multiple effects of caffeine on simulated high-intensity team-sport performance. Med Sci Sports Exerc 2005;37(11):1998–2005.

[94] Keisler BD, Hosey RG. Ergogenic aids: an update on ephedra. Curr Sports Med Rep 2005; 4:231–5.

[95] Berman JA, Setty A, Steiner MJ, et al. Complicated hypertension related to the abuse of ephedrine and caffeine alkaloids. J Addict Dis 2006;25(3):45–8.

[96] Calfee R, Fadale P. Popular ergogenic drugs and supplements in young athletes. Pediatrics 2006;117(3):e577–89.

[97] Fugh-Berman A, Myers A. Citrus aurantium, an ingredient of dietary supplements marketed for weight loss: current status of clinical and basic research. Exp Biol Med 2004; 229:698–704.

[98] Haaz S, Fontaine KR, Cutter G, et al. Citrus aurantium and synephrine alkaloids in the treatment of overweight and obesity: an update. Obes Rev 2006;7:79–88.

[99] Bouchard NC, Howland MA, Greller HA, et al. Ischemic stroke associated with use of an ephedra-free dietary supplement containing synephrine. Mayo Clin Proc 2005;80(4):541–5.

[100] Gange CA, Madias C, Felix-Getzik EM, et al. Variant angina associated with bitter orange in a dietary supplement. Mayo Clin Proc 2006;81(4):545–8.

[101] Sultan S, Spector J, Mitchell RM. Ischemic colitis associated with use of a bitter orange-containing dietary weight-loss supplement. Mayo Clin Proc 2006;81(12):1630–1.

[102] Requena B, Zabala M, Padial P, et al. Sodium bicarbonate and sodium citrate: ergogenic aids? J Strength Cond Res 2005;19(1):213–24.

[103] Oöpik V, Saaremets I, Medijainen L, et al. Effects of sodium citrate ingestion before exercise on endurance performance in well trained college runners. Br J Sports Med 2003;37: 485–9.

[104] Douroudos II, Fatouros IG, Gourgoulis V, et al. Dose-related effects of prolonged NaHCO$_3$ ingestion during high-intensity exercise. Med Sci Sports Exerc 2006;38(10): 1746–53.

[105] Bishop D, Claudius B. Effects of induced metabolic alkalosis on prolonged intermittent-sprint performance. Med Sci Sports Exerc 2005;37(5):759–67.

[106] Price M, Moss P, Rance S. Effects of sodium bicarbonate ingestion on prolonged intermittent exercise. Med Sci Sports Exerc 2003;35(8):1303–8.

[107] Bates N. Poisoning: sodium chloride and sodium bicarbonate. Emerg Nurse 2003;11(2): 33–7.

[108] Ganio MS, Casa DJ, Armstrong LE, et al. Evidence-based approach to lingering hydration questions. Clin Sports Med 2007;26:1–16.

[109] Kavouras SA, Armstrong LE, Maresh CM. Rehydration with glycerol: endocrine, cardio-vascular, and thermoregulatory responses during exercise in the heat. J Appl Physiol 2006; 100:442–50.

[110] Zoller H, Vogel W. Iron supplementation in athletes: first do no harm. Nutrition 2004;20: 615–9.

[111] Vincent JB. The potential value and toxicity of chromium picolinate as a nutritional supplement, weight loss agent and muscle development agent. Sports Med 2003;33(3):213–30.

[112] Kandel DB. Does marijuana use cause the use of other drugs? JAMA 2003;289:482–3.

ELSEVIER
SAUNDERS

PEDIATRIC CLINICS
OF NORTH AMERICA

Pediatr Clin N Am 54 (2007) 761–769

The History of the Development of Anabolic-Androgenic Steroids

Jennifer L. Dotson, MD[a,*], Robert T. Brown, MD[b,c]

[a]Department of Pediatrics, Columbus Children's Hospital, 700 Children's Drive,
Columbus, OH 43205, USA
[b]The Ohio State University College of Medicine, Columbus, OH, USA
[c]Section of Adolescent Health, Columbus Children's Hospital, 700 Children's Drive,
Columbus, OH 43205, USA

Anabolic-androgenic steroids (AASs) are synthetic derivatives of testosterone. The term "androgenic" indicates masculinizing. Androgens are responsible for stimulating the growth of the male reproductive tract and secondary sex characteristics. The term "anabolic" indicates tissue building and is the component of a steroid which is responsible for thickening of the vocal cords, enlargement of larynx, increasing libido, linear growth acceleration before epiphyseal plate closure, increasing muscle bulk and strength through dose-dependent hypertrophy, and decreasing body fat [1–3]. The anabolic action is mediated by androgen receptors on skeletal muscle [2]. Testosterone increases muscle protein synthesis, thus increasing the cross-sectional area of the fibers themselves, as well as increasing the myonuclear number [2,3].

The history of AASs is a tale that has its roots in ancient "endocrinology." More than 6000 years ago, farmers noted an enhanced ability to domesticate animals after castration. Years later, the medical theories of "humoralism" developed. This doctrine was based on a theory that attempted to explain diseases based on imbalances among the four humors: sanguine, choleric, melancholic, and phlegmatic [4]. In addition, ancient Egyptians and Romans believed that testicles and animal penises held special healing powers [1]. Ancient Greek athletes used a wide variety of alleged performance-enhancing drugs, such as plant extracts and testicular extracts. These early theories and practices marked the beginning of future discoveries.

---

* Corresponding author.
 E-mail address: dotsonj@chi.osu.edu (J.L. Dotson).

0031-3955/07/$ - see front matter © 2007 Elsevier Inc. All rights reserved.
doi:10.1016/j.pcl.2007.04.003
pediatric.theclinics.com

John Hunter (1728–1793) was a Scottish surgeon who was later appointed as Surgeon General for the British army. He made many noteworthy contributions to science, including contributions to the understanding of digestion, fetal development, venereal diseases, dentistry, and lymphatics. He conducted the first testicular transplant in 1786 in which he removed a testicle from a rooster and implanted it into a hen.

It was not until 1849 that Arnold Adolf Berthold (1803–1861) found evidence of a "bloodstream substance" from roosters that affected their appearance and behavior. His theory was correct. but it was not widely accepted by his contemporaries. Berthold was a professor at the University of Göttingen, and he performed experiments on roosters while he was a curator at a local zoo. He observed the impacts of castration and the reimplantation of testicular tissues on roosters. Once castrated, the roosters' combs decreased in size, they lost interest in the hens, and they lost their aggressive male behaviors. Those effects were reversed after reimplanting testicular tissues or extract, despite denervation [4,5]. Despite these findings, other researchers did not cite Berthold's work for nearly 50 years.

Perhaps the most well-known researcher of anatomy and physiology was Charles Edouard Brown-Sequard (1817–1894). Brown-Sequard, a prominent French physiologist and Harvard professor, was one of the founders of modern endocrinology [4]. He had a strong interest in endocrinology, and he studied adrenal glands, testes, thyroid, pancreas, liver, spleen, and kidneys. He is probably most famous for his auto-experimentation with testicular substances (extracted from guinea pigs and dogs), the results of which were published in 1889 [1,4]. He reported increased strength, mental abilities, and appetite and even claimed that the process relieved constipation and increased the arc of his urine stream [1]. Although no one is sure why he experienced these effects [5], his experiment caused others to investigate the testicular substance as a possible cure for various ailments, such as diabetes, tuberculosis, epilepsy, paralysis, gangrene, anemia, influenza, arteriosclerosis, Addison's disease, hysteria, and migraine headaches. He encouraged testing of his testosterone products by providing free samples to physicians [1]. Unfortunately, with such widespread use, shoddy researchers subjected animals and humans alike to high risks for infection and inflammation [4].

Austrian physiologist Oskar Zoth was the first person to propose injecting athletes with a hormonal substance, as published in his 1896 paper describing how the use of an "extract" improved muscular strength and the "neuromuscular apparatus," thus potentially improving athletic performance [1]. He and his physician partner, Fritz Pregl (1869–1930), self-injected testosterone extracts from bulls and measured the strength of their middle fingers by plotting them on "fatigue curves" [1]. They won the Nobel Prize in chemistry in 1923.

Substances referred to as "chemical messengers" were discovered in 1902 by English physiologists and professors, William Maddock Bayliss

(1860–1924) and Ernest Henry Starling (1866–1927), at University College London. Bayliss' research team was the focus of an animal rights controversy in 1903—the Brown Dog Affair—in which Bayliss was alleged to have performed a live dissection of a brown dog in his laboratory. He, of course, denied the accusation and won a civil suit, donating the money to the University for further research; he even wrote articles promoting the humane treatment of animals. Other accomplishments included contributions on shock, digestive system, and endocrinology; being knighted in 1922; and authoring four editions of *Principles of General Physiology*. Starling officially coined the term "hormone" in 1905 when giving a Croonian Lecture (prestigious lectureships) titled "The Chemical Control of the Functions of the Body" to the Royal College of Physicians [1,4–6]. The term "hormone" means "to urge on" or "impulse or arouse" in the sense of "to set in motion" in Greek. Years later, reports suggested that a Cambridge physiologist, William B. Hardy, actually suggested the term "hormone" to Bayliss and Starling. In 1911, Andre Pezard first noted a direct relationship between the amount of testicular extract injected into a rooster and the size of his comb [1].

An Austrian physician, Eugen Steinach (1861–1944), developed the "Steinach operation," an "autoplastic" treatment for the "middle-aged and listless" [4]. The 20-minute operation involved ligation of the vas deferens, often at the most proximal position to the testicle. This allegedly increased testosterone production. He believed that the incision produced a "back pressure" on the testicle, thus increasing testosterone production by the interstitial cells. He also implanted testicular tissue grafts between the peritoneal muscles. He reported that his patients were able to regrow hair, had better erections with less premature ejaculation, and had increased libido. Despite little clinical evidence of his claims on "rejuvenation," the results of his operations, at best, likely were due to the power of suggestion; however, he performed this procedure on some famous patients, including Sigmund Freud and William Butler Yeats. He also discovered, by transplanting male sex glands into females and vice versa, that guinea pigs developed sexual behaviors of the opposite sex. Later research proved that sex hormone injections have no effect on sexual orientation but that high doses of testosterone may increase sexual desire.

In 1913 in Chicago, Victor D. Lespinasse (1878–1923), a urologist, claimed that he cured a patient who had sexual dysfunction by transplanting a testicle from a donor. He removed the organ, made three transverse slices, and inserted them into muscle tissue around the patient's scrotum. His most famous patient was Harry F. McCormick (husband of Edith Rockefeller), whose case was described in *The New York Times*. Five years later, the first journal of *Endocrinology* was published.

In the 1920s, Sergio Voronoff, a Russian-French physician and surgeon, made a fortune from removing testes from animals (including the controversial monkey and chimpanzee gland transplants by way of vivisection, sparking campaigns from animal rights groups and satirical cartoons and books on the subject) and transplanting them into men. The chimpanzee tissue was not implanted inside the scrotum but instead in the tunica vaginalis. He concluded that his experiments with testicular transplants helped to relieve pain and provided a sense of well-being [1,5].

It was apparent to researchers that some substance circulating in the blood was responsible for their findings; however, it was not until 1929, when a German chemist and professor, Adolf Butenandt (1903–1995), isolated the first sex hormone, that a new path of discovery was initiated. He isolated estrone from the urine of pregnant women and later isolated 15 mg of androsterone ("andro" = male, "ster" = sterol, "one" = ketone) from 15,000 L of urine from local policemen [4]. Over the next few years, researchers found that the hormones isolated from the testes were more androgenic than were those isolated from urine [1]. Perhaps the most famous, and perhaps unethical, research of "organotherapy" occurred in the 1920s and 1930s at San Quentin prison in California where Leo Stanley transplanted the testicles from executed prisoners into impotent prisoners. He had a limited supply, so he turned to substituting a variety of animal gonads (from ram, sheep, goat, deer, and boar) to treat men who suffered from senility, epilepsy, and paranoia [1,4]. Over the years he performed hundreds of operations [1].

During the 1930s, three pharmaceutical companies each hired research teams to isolate the testicular hormone. The term testosterone ("testo" = testes, "ster" = sterol, "one" = ketone) was coined in 1935 by Karoly David and his research team [7]. Ernst Laqueur isolated testosterone from bull testes [5]. The research team was funded by the pharmaceutical company Organon in Oss, The Netherlands [4]. Later that same year (on a team funded by Schering Corporation in Berlin, Germany), Butendant and Gunicr Hanisch published "A Method for Preparing Testosterone from Cholesterol" in a German journal. Only a week later, Leopold Ruzicka (who synthesized androsterone in 1934) and A. Wettstein published "On the Artificial Preparation of the Testicular Hormone Testosterone (Andro-sten-3-one-17-ol)" in *Helvetica Chimica Acta* and applied for a patent. Butenandt and Ruzicka won the Nobel Prize for chemistry in 1939 [1,4]. Butenandt spent a large part of his career studying the sex hormones and their relationship with one another. His work laid the foundation for the production of cortisone.

In the late 1930s, experimentation using humans involved testosterone propionate (slow-release derivative) and methyl testosterone (oral form that was slower to metabolize). Most of the research at that time was focused on treating hypogonadism in men (inducing and maintaining secondary sexual characteristics and treating impotence) [1]. Charles D. Kochakian discovered an increase in protein anabolic processes, thus opening the door for the treatment of a variety of disorders by restoring tissue and stimulating growth [1].

In 1939, it was reported that daily topical application of testosterone by females enlarged the clitoris and increased sexual desire. The use of synthetic testosterone skyrocketed after publication of the book *The Male Hormone* by Paul de Kruif in 1945, which made claims of increasing libido and boosting athletic performance [1,4]. Testosterone was a proposed treatment for menorrhagia, dysmenorrhea, estrogen-derived breast cancers, and other breast conditions. It was reported to help relieve pain, increase appetite, and promote a "sense of well being." Despite these claims, physicians remained reluctant to begin widespread use among women because of the virilizing side effects [1]. Most of the profits from sale of this substance were obtained by way of the black market [1].

Body builders and athletes began using testosterone to increase muscle mass and to intensify training protocols on the West Coast of the United States in the late 1940s and early 1950s. The US Food and Drug Administration approved methandrostenolone in 1958. In the 1950s, Soviet Union and East German Olympic athletes were using AASs. They later found their way into the hands of Olympic competitors, including track and field athletes from many countries [1].

Paul Niehans wrote the 1960 book *Introduction to Cellular Therapy*, in which the main emphasis was on testicular secretions. He believed that testicle cell injections increased testosterone derivative excretion. Some of Paul Niehans' famous patients included Pope Pius XII, Bernard Baruch, and Aristotle Onassis [4]. In 1974, the International Olympic Committee banned the use of testosterone and its derivatives. AASs were widely abused in a variety of sports, including volleyball, cycling, swimming, soccer, and bobsledding.

Testosterone was studied using different forms. Scientists quickly learned it was ineffective, and even toxic (like 17 alpha-methyl testosterone), when taken orally; instead, it was synthesized into tiny pellets that were inserted subcutaneously. Longer-acting injectable forms of testosterone were synthesized in the 1950s (ie, testosterone enanthate). Over the following decade, the hormone was modified into derivatives that possessed more anabolic qualities [5].

In the 1970s, oral testosterone undecanoate was synthesized; however, it did not fare well in the oral form because of hepatic clearance and hepatotoxicity. Transdermal scrotal patches were derived in the 1990s. These allowed physiologic levels of testosterone to be acquired. Nonscrotal skin patches were developed, and testosterone gels were marketed. Today, there are short-acting buccal forms as well as the long-acting injectable testosterone undecanoate [5].

By the early 1990s, several pharmaceutical companies had stopped producing AASs. It was about at this time that the black market sales of AASs and counterfeit products increased secondary to the ease of Internet shopping and availability. Authentic steroids, as well as placebos and unpurified forms, were sold and abused. The US Congress placed anabolic steroids into the schedule III category of the Controlled Substance Act (CSA) in the Anabolic Steroid Control Act of 1990. This act included testosterone and all related chemical or pharmacologic substances that promoted muscle growth. Corticosteroids, progestins, and estrogens were not included in this act. The Anabolic Steroid Act of 1994 was an amendment to the CSA. It placed anabolic steroids as well as their precursors on the controlled substance list. Possession of the drugs without a prescription was now a federal crime. Studies of the effects of supplemental testosterone on aging men in the 1990s suggested an increase in word memory, special cognition, increased libido, decreased bone resorption, and increased lean body mass and strength [1]. McKinlay reported in the *Journal of Urology* that testosterone does not treat impotence [1]. In theory, prostatic tissue, including cancer and benign prostatic hypertrophy, can be stimulated by testosterone, but no compelling evidence has been reported that suggests an increased risk [8,9].

In summary, testosterone is produced in several areas within the human body. In men, most of it is synthesized in the Leydig cells of testes and in the adrenal glands; in women, testosterone is produced in the ovaries and adrenal glands, with a smaller fraction produced in other peripheral sites. Its synthesis involves a cholesterol precursor and a series of enzymatic reactions. Secretion is determined by a negative feedback mechanism that involves the anterior pituitary gland. It is here that luteinizing hormone (LH) and follicle-stimulating hormone are stored [4]. Elevated levels of testosterone affect the hypothalamus and pituitary. At high levels of testosterone, LH tends to be reduced (affecting sperm and endogenous testosterone production). Studies by the World Health Organization examined the use of anabolic steroids as a form of male birth control, but the results were not promising [1].

The evolution of the history of testosterone therapies is as interesting as the history of its development. Erectile dysfunction is one of the most researched ailments treated with testosterone, although any positive effects are questionable. In men with absent to low circulating levels of testosterone, treatment with testosterone increased libido, improved erectile function, and helped to maintain secondary sexual characteristics. In men with normal or mild hypotestosteronemia, studies have not shown consistent response to therapy. Those treated were reported to have increased sexual interest, increased arousal, increased frequency of intercourse, and nocturnal erections. In the early twentieth century, there was much interest in the hormonal influence of testosterone on sexuality and sexual preferences. It even was prescribed to "treat" homosexuals because it was theorized that male homosexuals had higher estrogen levels [4].

Testosterone has even played an important role in various ailments affecting women, such as treatment for some metastatic breast cancers [4,8]. Approximately one third of breast cancers are hormone dependent and respond to androgen therapies [1]. Other uses for testosterone are as postmenopausal hormone replacement therapy, for sexual dysfunction (by increasing libido), and for increasing bone density [8]. Only a small percentage of doctors in the United States prescribe testosterone creams to increase libido in women; this practice seems to be more popular in England and Australia [1].

Testosterone has been used to treat a variety of wasting conditions from HIV infection, posttrauma, including surgery and burns, and even after detainment in concentration camps [1,8]. Some clinical case studies showed an increase in appetite, lean muscle mass, and strength and an improved overall sense of well-being. Before the use of erythropoietin and bone marrow transplants, testosterone was used to help treat anemia (ie, chronic renal failure/hemodialysis) [1]. Psychiatrists prescribed anabolic steroids from the 1930s to the 1980s to treat psychoses, depression, and melancholia. Testosterone has been used as an adjunct in people with growth hormone deficiency or in boys with pubertal delay [1,8]. It even has been used in patients who had prostate disease and cardiovascular disease [8].

Essentially, there are three types of testosterone: endogenous, synthetic, and synthetic derivatives. AASs are discussed elsewhere in this issue. AASs are available legally only by prescription from a doctor, and sometimes they are used by veterinarians; they are found most often on the black market, typically smuggled into the United States from other countries (most commonly from Europe, Mexico, or Thailand), manufactured in clandestine facilities, or even by way of illegal pharmacy transportation. The black market forms are dangerous; the quality frequently is compromised by chemical substitutions in production and dilution. Often, steroids are purchased at gyms or by way of the Internet or mail order. Typically, AASs have a higher anabolic to androgenic ratio.

Frequently, abusers take AASs by "stacking," which means they take two or more at a time, sometimes even mixed them with stimulants or analgesics. Commonly, AASs are used cyclically, often "pyramiding." Low doses are increased gradually over a 6- to 12-week period and then decreased gradually over the second half of the cycle. This may be followed by a drug-free training period. Those who participate in pyramiding believe that it helps them to adjust to the high-dose AASs and allows the body to adjust hormonally during the drug-free cycle. Despite a lack of scientific evidence, users believe that they will see greater effects by "stacking" and "pyramiding" the drugs [9].

It is estimated that more than 1 million Americans abuse AASs, including many high school and college athletes [1,10]. A study survey conducted by the National Institute on Drug Abuse in 2004 reported that approximately 1.5% (down from 3% in 1999) of high school seniors admitted to using AASs [9]. It is difficult to estimate the true prevalence of abuse, perhaps because of the unwillingness of athletes to admit to using illegal drugs. AASs are banned by most sports organizations, including the International Olympic Committee.

Anabolic steroids possess a large side effect profile, including hepatotoxicity (including jaundice, cancer, and cystic lesions called peliosis hepaticus), hypercoagubility, hypertension, left ventricular hypertrophy, acne, hyper-cholesterolemia with increased low-density lipoprotein and decreased high-density lipoprotein, as well as an increased risk for cerebrovascular accident and acute myocardial infarction to name a few. Other risks include those that are associated with sharing needles, such as hepatitis B and C, HIV/AIDS, endocarditis, and local pain and abscess formations [9–12].

Steroid abuse among adolescents also can lead to precocious puberty and premature closure of their growth plates, resulting in stunted adult height secondary to premature epiphyseal closure. In men, side effects include dys-uria, baldness, gynecomastia, testicular atrophy, decreased sperm produc-tion, and even infertility. In women, side effects include masculinization, decreased body fat and breast size, hair loss, and clitoral enlargement. Nu-merous studies have linked aggression to high-dose steroid abuse, which in-creases the likelihood of fighting, physical and sexual abuse, vandalism, and burglary [9,10,13,14]. AAS withdrawal can lead to restlessness, insomnia, decreased libido, headaches, arthralgias, myalgias, fatigue, decreased appe-tite, depression, and even suicide [9–11].

The history of the development of AASs and their abuse for performance enhancement stem from ancient endocrinology thousands of years ago and spans to the present time of ongoing breakthrough research studies.

Acknowledgments

Special thanks to Dr. Peter Rogers for giving me this opportunity to write one of the articles and to Dr. Robert Brown who worked diligently with me as a coauthor and mentor.

Further readings

Center for Substance Abuse Research. Anabolic steroids. Available at: http://www.cesar.umd.edu/cesar/drugs/steroids.asp. Accessed February 12, 2007.
Eaton D, Kann L, Kinchen S, et al. Youth risk behavior survey—United States 2005. MMWR Surveillance Summaries. 2006;55(SS05):1–108.
Gomez JE. Performance-enhancing substances in adolescent athletes. Tex Med 2002;98:41–6.
Haupt HA, Revere GD. Anabolic steroids: a review of literature. Am J Sports Med 1984;12(6):469–84.
Kuhn C. Anabolic steroids. Recent Prog Horm Res 2002;57:411–30.
National Institute of Drug Abuse. Drugs of abuse information. Available at: http://www.nida.nih.gov/drugpages.html. Accessed February 12, 2007.
Parkinson A, Evans NA. Anabolic androgenic steroids: a survey of 500 users. Med Sci Sports Exerc 2006;38(4):644–51.

References

[1] Hoberman JM, Yesalis CE. The history of synthetic testosterone. Sci Am 1995;272:76–81.
[2] Sheffield-Moore M, Urban RJ, Wolf SE, et al. Short-term oxandrolone administration stimu-lates net muscle protein synthesis in young men. J Clin Endocrinol Metab 1999;84(8):2705–11.

[3] Bhasin S, Storer TW, Berman N, et al. The effects of supraphysiologic doses of testosterone on muscle size and strength in normal men. N Engl J Med 1996;335(1):1–7.
[4] Freeman ER, Bloom DA, McGuire EJ. A brief history of testosterone. J Urol 2001;165(2): 371–3.
[5] Nieschlag E. The history of testosterone [abstract]. Endocrine 2005;10:S2.
[6] Henriksen JH. Ernest Henry Starling (1866–1927): the scientist and the man. J Med Biogr 2005;13(1):22–30.
[7] David KG, Dingemanse E, Freud J, et al. On crystalline male hormone from testicles (testosterone). Hoppe Seylers Z Physiol Chem 1935;233:281.
[8] Margo K, Winn R. Testosterone treatments: why, when and how? Am Fam Physician 2006; 73(9):1591–8.
[9] Anabolic Steroid abuse. Available at: http://www.steroidabuse.gov/. Accessed February 12, 2007.
[10] Evans NA. Current concepts in anabolic-androgenic steroids. Am J Sports Med 2004;32: 534–42.
[11] United States Anti-Doping Agency. Available at: http://www.usantidoping.org/. Accessed February 12, 2007.
[12] Dhal R, Stout CW, Link MS, et al. Cardiovascular toxicities of performance-enhancing substances in sports. Mayo Clin Proc 2005;80(10):1307–15.
[13] Choi PY, Parrott AC, Cowan D. High-dose anabolic steroids in strength athletes: effects upon hostility and aggression. Hum Psychopharmacol 1990;5(4):349–56.
[14] Moss HB, Panzak GL, Tarter RE. Personality, mood and psychiatric symptoms among anabolic steroid users. Am J Addict 1992;1(4):315–24.

PEDIATRIC CLINICS
OF NORTH AMERICA

Pediatr Clin N Am 54 (2007) 771–785

Anabolic-Androgenic Steroids: Use and Abuse in Pediatric Patients

Julie M. Kerr, MD[a,b,*], Joseph A. Congeni, MD[a,b]

[a]Northeastern Ohio Universities College of Medicine, 4209 State Route 44, PO Box 95,
Rootstown, OH 44272, USA
[b]Division of Sports Medicine, Akron Children's Hospital, Sports Medicine Center,
388 South Main Street, Suite 207, Akron, OH 44311, USA

The "win at all costs" mentality fuels athletes to seek performance-enhancing substances, such as anabolic-androgenic steroids (AASs), to gain an advantage over their opponents. Nonathletes espouse this same attitude to "win" the battle of attractiveness. They view AASs as the means to achieving what they believe is a more desirable muscular physique. These beliefs have filtered from professional, Olympic, and collegiate levels into high schools, middle schools, and grade schools. An enhanced understanding of AASs and the motivations behind their abuse will arm the pediatrician with the ability to engage one's patients in a balanced discussion of the benefits and costly risks of AASs and successfully deter further use.

History

High levels of AAS abuse have been attributed to professional football players, bodybuilders, weight lifters, and track and field throwers since the 1960s. The exceptional athletic performance of the East German female swimmers in the 1976 Montreal Olympics brought further public attention to AAS athletic use. It was not until the 1980s, however, that the medical community admitted that these substances were effective [1]. Since that time, the pervasive use of AASs by professional athletes has garnered significant media attention, culminating most recently in the ongoing investigation of the use of illegal performance enhancing drugs by some of baseball's top players. *Juiced*, a book by Jose Canseco, details his steroid use and the widespread use of anabolic steroids in Major League Baseball.

---

* Corresponding author. Division of Sports Medicine, Akron Children's Hospital, Sports Medicine Center, 388 South Main Street, Suite 207, Akron, OH 44311.
E-mail address: jkerr@chmca.org (J.M. Kerr).

0031-3955/07/$ - see front matter © 2007 Elsevier Inc. All rights reserved.
doi:10.1016/j.pcl.2007.04.010   *pediatric.theclinics.com*

The fame achieved by such professional athletes may be what makes trying AASs so enticing to adolescents.

Physiology

Several studies have contributed to an enlarging body of evidence regarding the anabolic "tissue-building" effects of AASs on their primary target, skeletal muscle. The actions of AASs on the musculoskeletal system have been shown to influence lean body mass, muscle size and strength, protein metabolism, bone metabolism, and collagen synthesis [2–8]. Over a period of 10 to 20 weeks, a supraphysiologic dose of testosterone administered to healthy young men can increase lean body mass, as well as muscle size and strength with or without exercise [2,3,8]. These significant increases are dose dependent and only occur with doses of 300 mg per week and higher [3,8]. The most profound effects are noted when supraphysiologic doses accompany a training program and are used in conjunction with a diet adequate in protein and calories [2,9,10].

Testosterone-induced muscle hypertrophy and increases in muscle strength are the result of increases in the cross-sectional area of muscle fibers and myonuclear number [8]. Research suggests that these anabolic effects are mediated by testosterone-influenced increases in muscle protein synthesis, creating a positive nitrogen balance [5,7,11]. Androgen receptors in skeletal muscle regulate the transcription of the target genes that control the accumulation of DNA needed for muscle growth. Complementary effects include glucocorticoid antagonism, which minimizes the catabolic actions of corticosteroids released during the stress of athletic activity. Similarly, stimulation of the growth hormone insulin-like growth factor-1 axis [12] and enhanced collagen synthesis and bone mineral density [13] are additional anabolic effects.

AASs induce a state of euphoria and diminished fatigue that enables prolongation of training sessions by users. Recent data may explain how AASs exert these psychoactive effects on the brain. Henderson and colleagues [14] proposed that AAS-mediated acute and chronic changes in the gamma-aminobutyric acid (GABA) receptor system cause many of the known behavioral effects. For instance, the immediate effects of decreased anxiety and enhanced sense of well-being that are experienced by AAS users likely arise from enhancement of forebrain GABAergic circuits. In contrast, anxiety and aggression are the result of a down-regulation of GABA receptor expression secondary to chronic AAS exposure. Further study may reveal that expression of these behaviors is influenced by the age and gender of the AAS user and the particular chemical composition of the AAS administered.

Clinical uses

The anabolic properties of AASs have proven beneficial for some therapeutic applications. They have been used in clinical practice since the 1940s for the treatment of trauma, burns, extensive surgery, radiation therapy, and chronic debilitating illnesses [15–18]. Before the advent of bone marrow transplantation and synthetic erythropoietin, AASs were used often in the treatment of various types of anemias. AASs have shown promise in treating short stature, as in Turner's syndrome, or constitutional growth and puberty delay. Since 1985, the clinical use of AASs has increased 400%, mostly due to the management of AIDS-associated wasting syndrome. AASs may enhance the effects of the increased caloric intake and exercise regimen [19]. A pilot study in malnourished HIV-infected children as young as 4 years old showed that oxandrolone treatment was well-tolerated and improved nutritional status. After 3 months of treatment, the study subjects experienced an accelerated rate of weight gain, increased body mass index, increased muscle mass, and decreased fat stores as compared with pretreatment values. The results were supported further by the improved serum albumin levels noted during the course of treatment. Future studies using a larger study population and longer- or higher-dose AAS administration would strengthen the current data [20]. In patients with severe burns, AASs may play an important role in reversing the catabolic state. A small prospective randomized study of patients who had burns showed that those receiving oxandrolone in addition to a high-protein diet experienced a significantly greater increase in weight and physical therapy index than did patients who were treated with diet alone [21]. AAS therapy seems to be promising in the treatment of malnutrition and muscle wasting seen in patients who have end-stage renal disease. In addition to the increase in lean body mass, these patients also benefit from a stimulated erythropoiesis resulting from the administration of AASs [22,23]. Such positive effects warrant further study [19].

Legal issues

The nonmedical use of AASs has been banned by the International Olympic Committee, the United States Olympic Committee, and the National Collegiate Athletic Association. Such use also is denounced by the American Medical Association, the American College Health Association, the American Academy of Pediatrics, the American College of Sports Medicine, and the National Strength and Conditioning Association [24]. Steroids are banned from use by all major sporting leagues, although each has its own testing and penalization policies [25]. The US Federal Government and most state governments have enacted laws regarding the distribution, possession, or prescription of AASs. The Federal Food, Drug, and Cosmetic Act was amended as part of the 1988 Anti-Drug Abuse act, such that distribution of AASs or possession with intent to distribute without a valid prescription became a felony. Such offenses are punishable by a prison term of up to 5 years or fines totaling $250,000 [25]. In 1990, the

Anabolic Steroids Control Act was signed into law, thereby classifying AASs as Schedule III drugs within the Controlled Substances Act. The Drug Enforcement Agency now controls the manufacture, importation, exportation, distribution, and dispensing of AASs [26].

Sources

Despite the above-mentioned barriers, AASs are still making their way into the hands of adolescents and children. Most commonly, the sources are bodybuilding gyms that obtain the drugs by way of a multimillion dollar illicit black market: foreign mail order, Internet dealers, or Internet pharmacies [2]. Most concerning about such sources is that the purity and actual content of the product received cannot be guaranteed.

Prevalence of adolescent anabolic-androgenic steroid use

The first reported adolescent use of AASs was in 1959 by a high school football player [27]. Current estimates of high school steroid usage range from 4% to 11% in boys and up to 3.3% in girls [28,29]. The landmark study of prevalence that was performed by Buckley and colleagues [30] involved a nationwide survey of more than 3000 boys. They found that 6.6% of male high school seniors had tried steroids, with 67% initiating use by 16 years of age and 40% using multiple cycles. These results have been confirmed in later studies of Indiana high school football players documenting a 6% use rate [31] and a 2003 Centers for Disease Control and Prevention report finding a 6.4% use of steroids by 12th-grade boys. The largest nationwide cohort of nearly 50,000 students is being examined in the Monitoring the Future study [32]. As of 2004, results of this ongoing study indicated a 1.3%, 2.3%, and 3.3% annual prevalence of male AAS users in the eighth, 10th, and 12th grades, respectively. Girls in the 12th grade had a 1.7% use rate in this study, whereas the Centers for Disease Control and Prevention reported a 3.3% lifetime prevalence in 12th-grade girls.

Prevalence studies have extended to middle school populations as well. A 1993 study of Modesto, California seventh-grade students was the first to document the use of steroids in students aged 12 to 15 years [33]. The overall rate of use reported was 3.8%, with more male students (4.7% versus 3.2% in female students) admitting to using AASs. A later article published data from a study of Massachusetts students between 9 and 13 years of age [34]. AAS use was reported by 2.7% of all middle school students surveyed, with 2.6% of boys and 2.8% of girls reporting use. As in other studies, the prevalence of AAS use increased with increasing age. Both of these regional studies were consistent with data from Yesalis [35], who reviewed AAS prevalence rates among junior high school students in the United States (2% for sixth graders and 2.3 to 3% for eighth graders).

AAS use by adolescents is not limited to the United States. Three Canadian studies, two Swedish surveys, two South African investigations, one British study, and one Australian investigation reported an overall prevalence range between 1% and 3%. Although slightly lower, these rates approximate those reported in the United States, demonstrating that the impact of AASs on athletic performance and physical appearance reaches across cultures [36].

Risk factors for adolescent anabolic-androgenic steroid abuse

Many studies of adolescent AAS users and abusers have attempted to create a profile of the typical user. The following discussion reviews some of the data relating to demographics, school performance, athletic participation, and personality of AAS users.

Demographic factors

Generally, the relative risk of AAS use is at least two to three times greater for male adolescents. The review of numerous studies shows a wide variation in the age range of AAS users. Race and ethnicity of AAS users is equally unclear. Some studies reported greater use among minorities [30,33,37–40], whereas others revealed a higher rate among white adolescents [41–46]. One regional study reported a significantly higher rate in blacks [33]. Other studies reported no racial difference in adolescent AAS use. Likewise, no clear-cut relationship exists regarding geographic location, city size, or school size.

Academic factors

There may be some association between AAS use and poor academic performance. In a large national study, DuRant and colleagues [47] stated that students who reported below-average academic performance had a significantly higher prevalence of AAS use than did average or above-average students; however, two studies, reported no relationship between academic achievement and AAS use [48,49]. Future studies regarding this question are needed.

Athletic performance

Adolescents use AASs as a method to improve their athletic performance. AAS users are significantly more likely than are nonusers to participate in school-sponsored athletic programs [30,40,50–53]. Sports requiring muscular strength and power are those most closely associated with AAS use among their participants. Such sports include football, wrestling, and track and field [30,40,41,50,51,54–56]. Faigenbaum and colleagues [34] reported greater AAS use in gymnastics and weight training in their study sample. Strength undoubtedly is an asset to gymnasts, and, thus, correlates well with the observed higher percentage; however, they were concerned with the suggestion that some young gymnasts may use AASs to stunt their growth because they believe that small stature confers an advantage in gymnastics. It is important to realize that approximately 30% to 40% of adolescent AAS users do not participate in a school-sponsored sport. These users likely participate in bodybuilding or weightlifting activities [30,40].

Personality and behavioral factors

A considerable percentage of adolescents turn to AAS use to help them achieve an attractive physique. This is the second most popular reason for using AASs. One study of bodybuilders suggests that the drive for a muscular physique sometimes reaches an unhealthy extreme and likens the use of AAS to the "unhealthy extremes" that are characteristic of anorexic and bulimic individuals. Just as eating disordered women see their bodies as larger than they actually are, some men perceive themselves as smaller than they actually are. Taylor [57] refers to this phenomenon as "bigamerexia" and suggests that this misperception may be a contributory factor in AAS use. This misperception is likely evident in many ninth-grade boys, who—in the early stages of puberty—are impatient with their muscular development. Perceiving themselves smaller than their peers, these boys may engage in AAS use as a shortcut to increasing muscle strength and size [39]. Exposure to the media may intensify this body dysmorphia. Field and colleagues [58] examined this possibility in a study of supplement use among adolescents. They found that girls and boys who reported thinking frequently about wanting more defined muscles and those who were trying to emulate the look of same-gender figures in the media were more than three times more likely to use agents to build muscle or improve appearance.

Adolescent AAS use has been associated with the use of other harmful drugs, including cigarettes, smokeless tobacco, marijuana, alcohol, cocaine, and injected drugs. These behaviors support a risk behavior framework hypothesized by Jessor [59] in his Problem Behavior Theory. He proposed that there are intraindividual similarities among adolescent problem behaviors such that they cluster to form a "risk behavior syndrome." Thus, AAS use would be considered a part of this cluster rather than an isolated behavior. Middleman and colleagues [60] applied this theory to a study of Massachusetts high school AAS users. They noted that the frequency of AAS use was associated with driving after drinking alcohol, carrying a gun, sexual promiscuity, unprotected intercourse, injury in a fight requiring medical attention, history of a sexually transmitted disease, not wearing a helmet on a motorcycle, not wearing a passenger seatbelt, and a suicide attempt requiring medical attention. Another concerning health-compromising behavior is the sharing of needles and multidose vials by between 25% and 33% of adolescent AAS users. This practice contributes to the risk for acquiring infections, such as HIV, hepatitis B, and hepatitis C [61,62].

Dosage and patterns of use

Anabolic steroids may be taken orally or injected intramuscularly [63] and are grouped into three main classes [14]. Testosterone esters, such as testosterone propionate, are injected compounds and constitute class I. Class II agents include the nortestosterone derivatives (eg, nandrolone decanoate and nandrolone phenpropionate). Class I and II AASs exert effects at androgen receptors as well as at estrogen receptors by way of aromatization to estradiol [17]. The third class of AASs are those alkylated at C-17 and are the orally administered compounds oxymetholone, methandrostenolone, and stanozolol. Alkylation of these compounds involves the addition of a methyl or ethyl group to the carbon at position 17 of the steroid backbone. The alkylation slows the hepatic metabolism of these agents [19]. These and other common oral and injectable preparations are listed in Table 1.

A typical pattern of use consists of a combination of injectable and oral steroids taken during 6- to 12-week cycles. Injectable forms tend to be favored by users because they are less hepatotoxic than the oral forms [1]. Because oral

Table 1
More commonly abused anabolic steroids

Generic name	How supplied	Recommended dosage	Abused dosage[a]
Oxymetholone (O)	50 mg	1–5 mg/kg/d	50–100 mg/d
Oxandrolone (O)	2.5 mg	5–10 mg/d	15 mg/d
Nandrolone decanoate (I)	25 mg/mL, 5 mL	100–200 mg/wk	200–400 mg/wk
Methandrostenolone (O & I)	5 mg, 10 mg/mL	—	15–30 mg/d, 50–100 mg/wk
Boldenone undecyclenate (I)	50 mg/mL	—	5 mL/wk
Methenolone (O & I)	50 mg/ml; 50, 100 mg/mL	—	50–100 mg/d, 200 mg/wk
Testosterone propionate, phenyl propionate, isocaporate, decanoate (I)	250 mg/mL	—	250 mg/wk
Testosterone cypionate (I)	200 mg/mL	25–200 mg/wk	1–3 mL/wk
Testosterone enanthate (I)	200 mg/mL	25–200 mg/mL	1–3 mL/wk
Testosterone propionate (I)	100 mg/10 mL	50–150 mg/wk	200–400 mg/wk
Testosterone suspension (I)	100 mg/10 mL	—	50 mg/d
Stanozolol (O & I)	2 mg, 50 mg/mL	6 mg/d,	16–30 mg/d, 3–5 mL/wk

Abbreviations: O, oral; I, injectable.

[a] Abused dosages may vary greatly by gender, personal experience, availability of specific steroids, performance and appearance goals, and the simultaneous use of several steroids.

Data from Bahrke MS, Yesalis CE, Brower KJ. Anabolic-androgenic steroid abuse and performance-enhancing drugs among adolescents. Child Adolesc Psychiatr Clin N Am 1998;7(4):826.

preparations are cleared from the system more quickly, they are the preferred form of steroids when drug testing is anticipated. The simultaneous use of multiple steroids is referred to as "stacking." A pattern of increasing a dose through a cycle is called "pyramiding." Pyramiding can lead to doses 10 to 40 times greater than the dose recommended for medical indications. By stacking and pyramiding doses, the user hopes to maximize steroid receptor binding, thereby reducing toxic side effects. These patterns have remained popular, despite the lack of scientific evidence of a benefit [29]. Some users take other drugs concurrently in an effort to minimize side effects. These "accessory" medications include clomiphene and human chorionic gonadotropin and are administered to reverse the endogenous testosterone production. Additionally, tamoxifen and antiaromatase drugs can prevent or decrease gynecomastia by limiting estrogenic effects and the metabolism of excess testosterone derivatives to estradiol [63]. It is not uncommon for users to take other legal performance-enhancing substances and dietary supplements, such as creatine, glutamine, and protein, while using AASs [64].

Adverse effects

For years, scientists have attempted to dissociate the anabolic properties from the androgenic characteristics of AASs, to no avail. Therefore, both components exert adverse effects on various tissues and body systems.

Hepatic

Various studies have shown transient elevations in liver function tests in conjunction with AAS use [10,65,66]. The C-17 alkylated oral preparations are associated most often with liver toxicity [67]. Elevations in aspartate transaminase, alanine transaminase, lactate dehydrogenase, and alkaline phosphatase have been reported [10]. Values measured can be two to three times the normal range, peaking within 2 to 3 weeks of consumption. Usually, a return to baseline is seen within several weeks of discontinuation [68]. Many AAS users also abuse alcohol, thus compounding the hepatic adverse effects.

Anabolic-related cholestasis has been reported to occur in varying frequency from a few cases to up to 17.3% in some studies [69,70]. The transient jaundice that results is secondary to biliary stasis rather than structural hepatic injury. Structural lesions have been studied in case reports of the blood-filled cysts of peliosis hepatis [71]. Internal hemorrhage or hepatic failure can occur secondary to such lesions.

Hepatocellular adenomas have been associated with high-dose AAS, long periods of administration of AAS, or in AAS users with a predisposing medical condition [10,67]. It is particularly difficult to differentiate adenomas from hepatocellular carcinoma by ultrasound. Prompt identification of these lesions is critical because the potential for malignant transformation may increase if a late diagnosis is made [72].

Cardiovascular

Altered lipid profiles in AAS users are reflected in increased low-density lipoprotein and decreased high-density lipoprotein [66,71,73]. The oral C-17 alkylated steroids seem to exert the greatest effects on the lipid profile [68,74,75]. Thrombus formation has been postulated by way of these adverse lipid changes and is supported further by findings of AAS-induced increased platelet aggregation, enhanced coagulation enzyme activity, and coronary vasospasm [76].

Hypertension in AAS users has been reported and is likely the result of blood volume increases and fluid retention [71,76]. This effect, as well as the finding of increased septal thickness and left ventricular mass reported in AAS users [77,78], can lead to significant detrimental cardiac remodeling.

Reproductive/endocrine

Exogenous steroid administration provides feedback inhibition of luteinizing and follicle-stimulating hormones, which leads to testicular atrophy and decreased spermatogenesis. This testicular impairment is reversed upon cessation of AAS use. Excess steroids undergo peripheral aromatization to estrogens, which results in feminizing changes of high voice pitch and male gynecomastia [71]. In long-term AAS abuse, this gynecomastia is irreversible, leaving surgical correction as the only solution [79]. In addition to the female side effects of decreased menstruation and breast tissue atrophy, virilizing effects also occur and include deepened voice, clitoromegaly, and hirsutism. Sometimes these effects are irreversible, even after discontinuation of AAS use [80].

Musculoskeletal

Experimental evidence exists that the use of AASs combined with intense exercise can cause structural and biomechanical alterations of tendons resulting in rupture. Structurally, the collagen fibril alignment is highly disorganized. From a biomechanical perspective, when muscle strength is increased with AAS use, the tendon becomes stiffer, absorbs less energy, and is more likely to fail during physical activity [81].

Premature growth cessation due to physeal closure in younger users has not been studied systematically. Such case reports of the resultant permanent short stature have been described for several decades [82].

Dermatologic

Severe cases of acne, especially on the face and back of AAS users, are common dermatologic findings. Premature baldness is noted as well. Dickinson and colleagues [83] reported multiple cases of serious muscular abscesses resulting from the common practice of shared needles and shared steroid vials among adolescent AAS users. A limited knowledge of sterile injection technique, as well as limited access to sterile needles and syringes are likely additional causative factors in these infections.

Psychiatric

AAS use has been associated with self-reported changes in mood and behavior. A study by Pope and Katz [84] identified psychiatric syndromes in weightlifters using AASs. Twenty-three percent of AAS users experienced major mood changes of mania, hypomania, or major depression. Also common in AAS users was aggressive behavior resulting in fights, domestic disturbances, assaults, and arrests. Data from the National Household Survey on Drug Abuse have demonstrated a strong association between AAS use and self-acknowledged acts of violence against people and crimes against property [85]. In general, the behavioral effects of AASs are variable, short-lived on discontinuation, and seem to be related to the type and dosage of AAS.

The potential for physical dependence upon AASs does exist. In one study of AAS users, 50% of them met the *Diagnostic and Statistical Manual of Mental Disorders, Fourth Edition* criteria for dependence or abuse of steroids [86]. Physical symptoms of withdrawal are similar to those seen during alcohol and opioid withdrawal, including diaphoresis, myalgias, nausea, and increases in blood pressure and heart rate [87]. Withdrawal may also be characterized by depressive symptoms [88]. Deeply entrenched body dissatisfaction and body dysmorphic disorder may underlie a psychologic dependence. Clearly, the addictive potential of AASs cannot be discounted [89].

Prevention efforts

The implementation of drug-testing policies has been considered as a possible preventive strategy. Data from the National Federation of State High School Associations indicate, however, that only 13% of schools test athletes and, of those schools, only 29% test for AASs. The reasons for the low number of testing programs include financial constraints (~$120 per test) and the fact that testing often can be circumvented by the user. Dose titration with newer transdermal delivery systems of testosterone or discontinuation of use before a scheduled test can maintain levels below a testing threshold [90]. Testing only athletes also will miss a significant percentage of nonathlete users.

Educational programs have been suggested as a more effective means of deterring AAS use. Goldberg and colleagues [91] tested a team-based educational intervention designed to reduce Portland, Oregon high school football players' intent to use AASs. The Adolescents Training and Learning to Avoid Steroids Program consisted of 50-minute class sessions that were delivered over a 7-week period by coaches and athlete team leaders. The sessions combined drug education with attainment of personal skills to assist athletes in resisting the social influences that fuel an athlete's desire to use AASs. Athletes in this intervention group gained a greater knowledge of the consequences of AAS use, were more skeptical about the media's promotion of AASs, and had improved drug-refusal skills. These results are certainly encouraging and follow-up data are eagerly anticipated.

The pediatrician's office can be a valuable educational setting as well. Using "scare tactics" as a prevention effort to dissuade adolescents from becoming AAS users has been proven to weaken physician credibility and may even encourage use [92]. Rather, Metzl [93] offers the concept of "thoughtful discouragement" as the key to effective prevention. He recommends that the clinician first recognize that a patient may be using AASs. The sports preparticipation physical examination offers an ideal opportunity to note any physical changes suggestive of AAS use and to ask whether the patient is using a performance-enhancing substance. Education is the next step and should be a balanced discussion focusing on the current research, the physiologic effects, and the adverse events. A concerning trend in 12th graders showed a steadily decreasing perceived risk for steroid use yearly since 1993. Only 55% of seniors now consider steroid use as a great risk [32]. Finally, healthy alternatives to AAS use must be presented. A supervised strength-training program among children as young as 8 years of age is a safe and effective means of increasing strength and improving athletic performance [94]. By emphasizing repetitions rather than maximum weight lifting, baseline strength can be increased by 30% to 40% [95].

Summary

Our society equates success with winning. The drive to win athletic competitions or the obsession with achieving the perfect physique has made adolescents and children increasingly vulnerable to the lure of AASs. The increases in muscular size and strength that are characteristic of AASs occur with attendant short-term adverse effects and the potential for long-term health consequences. A mindset of invincibility that is typical of many adolescents allows them to be willing to pay the price of these negative events for the chance to gain a competitive edge.

Educational programs addressing the social, media, and peer influences that perpetuate adolescent use of AASs have shown promise in decreasing the intent to use. Such educational programs need to be directed toward middle school classrooms to decrease the rate of first use in this age group. Physician dissemination of accurate information to parents, coaches, and school administrators is vital to the creation of intervention programs. By demonstrating a knowledge base that earns adolescent respect, the pediatrician will be able to effectively discourage AAS use and convince the patient that there is no substitute for sound nutrition and a sensible strength-training program.

References

[1] Dawson RT. Drugs in sport—the role of the physician. J Endocrinol 2001;170:55–61.

[2] Bhasin S, Storer TW, Berman N, et al. The effects of supraphysiologic doses of testosterone on muscle size and strength in normal men. N Engl J Med 1996;335:1–6.

[3] Bhasin S, Woodhouse L, Casaburi R, et al. Testosterone dose-response relationships in healthy young men. Am J Physiol Endocrinol Metab 2001;281:E1172–81.

[4] Evans NA. Current concepts in anabolic-androgenic steroids. Am J Sports Med 2004;32: 534–42.

[5] Ferrando AA, Tipton KD, Doyle D, et al. Testosterone injection stimulates net protein synthesis but not tissue amino acid transport. Am J Physiol 1998;275:E864–71.

[6] Parssinin M, Karla T, Kovanen V, et al. The effect of supraphysiologic doses of anabolic androgenic steroids on collagen metabolism. Int J Sports Med 2000;21:406–11.

[7] Sheffield-Moore M, Urban RJ, Wolf SE, et al. Short-term oxandrolone administration stimulates net muscle protein synthesis in young men. J Clin Endocrinol Metab 1999;84:2705–11.

[8] Sinha-Hakim I, Artaza J, Woodhouse L, et al. Testosterone-induced increase in muscle size in healthy young men is associated with muscle fiber hypertrophy. Am J Physiol Endocrinol Metab 2002;283:E154–64.

[9] American College of Sports Medicine. Position statement on anabolic-androgenic steroids in sports. Med Sci Sports Exerc 1987;19:534–9.

[10] Haupt HA, Rovere GD. Anabolic steroids: a review of the literature. Am J Sports Med 1984; 12:469–84.

[11] Urban RJ, Bodenburg YH, Gilkison C, et al. Testosterone administration to elderly men increases skeletal muscle strength and protein synthesis. Am J Physiol 1995;269:E820–6.

[12] Kuhn CM. Anabolic steroids. Recent Prog Horm Res 2002;57:411–34.

[13] Bagatell CJ, Breamner WJ. Androgens in men—uses and abuses. N Engl J Med 1996;334: 707–14.

[14] Henderson LP, Penatti CAA, Jones BL, et al. Anabolic androgenic steroids and forebrain GABAergic transmission. Neuroscience 2006;138:793–9.

[15] Rosenfield RL. Role of androgens in growth and development of the fetus, child and adolescent. Adv Pediatr 1972;19:172–213.

[16] Pardridge WM. Serum bioavailability of sex steroid hormones. Clin Endocrinol Metab 1986; 15:259–78.

[17] Winters S. Androgens and anti-androgens. In: Brody TM, Larner J, Minneman KP, editors. Human pharmacology: molecular to clinical. 3rd edition. St. Louis (MO): Mosby; 1998. p. 519–31.

[18] Griffin JE, Wilson JD, et al. Disorders of the testes and the male reproductive tract. In: Wilson JD, Foster DW, Kronenberg HM, editors. Williams textbook of endocrinology. 9th edition. Philadelphia: Saunders; 1998. p. 839–76.

[19] Basaria S, Wahlstrom J, Dobs AS. Anabolic-androgenic steroid therapy in the treatment of chronic diseases. J Clin Endocrinol Metab 2001;86(11):5108–17.

[20] Fox-Wheeler S, Heller L, Salata CM, et al. Evaluation of the effects of oxandrolone on malnourished HIV-positive pediatric patients. Pediatrics 1999;104:73.

[21] Demling RH, DeSanti L. Oxandrolone, an anabolic steroid, significantly increases the rate of weight gain in the recovery phase after major burns. J Trauma 1997;27:46–51.

[22] Shahidi NT. Androgens and erythropoiesis. N Engl J Med 1973;289:72–80.

[23] Evans RP, Amerson AB. Androgens and erythropoiesis. J Clin Pharmacol 1974;14:94–101.

[24] Council on Scientific Affairs. Medical and nonmedical uses of anabolic-androgenic steroids. JAMA 1990;264:2923–7.

[25] Calfee R, Fadale P. Popular ergogenic drugs and supplements in young athletes. Pediatrics 2006;117:577–89.

[26] Yesalis CE, Bahrke MS. Anabolic-androgenic steroids. Current issues. Sports Med 1995; 19(5):326–40.

[27] Sturmi JE, Diorio DJ. Anabolic agents. Clin Sports Med 1998;17:283–97.
[28] Grunbaum JA, Kann L, Kinchen SA, et al. Youth risk behavior surveillance: United States, 2003. MMWR Surveill Summ 2004;53:1–96.
[29] American Academy of Pediatrics Committee on Sports Medicine and Fitness. Adolescents and anabolic steroids: a subject review. Pediatrics 1997;99:904–8.
[30] Buckley WE, Yesalis CE, Friedl KE, et al. Estimated prevalence of anabolic steroid use among male high school seniors. JAMA 1998;260:3441–5.
[31] Stilger VG, Yesalis CE. Anabolic-androgenic steroid use among high school football players. J Community Health 1999;24:131–45.
[32] US Department of Health and Human Services. Monitoring the future study: overview of key findings. 2004. Available at: www.monitoringthefuture.org. Accessed January 30, 2007.
[33] Radakovich J, Broderick P, Pickell G. Rate of anabolic-androgenic steroid use among students in junior high school. J Am Board Fam Pract 1993;6:341–5.
[34] Faigenbaum AD, Zaichkowsky LD, Gardner DE, et al. Anabolic steroid use by male and female middle school students. Pediatrics 1998;101:6.
[35] Yesalis CE, editor. Incidence of anabolic steroid use: a discussion of methodological issues Anabolic steroids in sport and exercise. Champaign (IL): Human Kinetic Publishers; 1993. p. 49–69.
[36] Bahrke MS, Yesalis CE, Kopstein AN, et al. Risk factors associated with anabolic-androgenic steroid use among adolescents. Sports Med 2000;29:397–405.
[37] Schwellnus M, Lambert M, Todd M, Juritz JM. Androgenic anabolic steroid use among matric pupils. A survey of the prevalence of use in the western Cape. S Afr Med J 1992;82:154–8.
[38] Handelsman DJ, Gupta L. Prevalence and risk factors for anabolic-androgenic steroid use in Australian high school students. Int J Androl 1997;20:159–64.
[39] DuRant RH, Ashworth CS, Newman C, et al. Stability of the relationship between anabolic steroid use and multiple substance use among adolescents. J Adolesc Health 1994;15(2): 111–6.
[40] DuRant RH, Rickert VI, Ashworth CS, et al. Use of multiple drugs among adolescents who use anabolic steroids. N Engl J Med 1993;328(13):922–6.
[41] Collins MA. Prevalence of anabolic steroid use among male and female high school students [abstract]. J Strength Cond Res 1993;7(4):251.
[42] Komoroski EM, Rickert VI. Adolescent body image and attitudes to anabolic steroid use. Am J Dis Child 1992;146:823–8.
[43] Milkow VA. Alcohol, tobacco, and other drug use by 9th-12th grade students: results from the 1993 North Carolina Youth Risk Behavior Survey. Raleigh (NC): North Carolina Department of Public Instruction; 1994.
[44] Texas Commission on Alcohol and Drug Abuse. 1994 Texas Scholl Survey of substance abuse among students: grades 7–12. Austin (TX): Texas Commission on Alcohol and Drug Abuse; 1995.
[45] Salva PS, Bacon GE. Anabolic steroids: interest among parents and nonathletes. South Med J 1991;84(5):552–6.
[46] South Carolina Department of Education and South Carolina Commission on Alcohol and Drug Abuse (1989–1990 and 1992–1993 School Years). The youth survey results regarding alcohol and other drug use in South Carolina. Columbia (SC): South Carolina Commission on Alcohol and Drug Abuse; 1994.
[47] DuRant RH, Escobedo LG, Heath GW. Anabolic-steroid use, strength training, and multiple drug use among adolescents in the United States. Pediatrics 1995;96:23–8.
[48] Adalf EM, Smart RG. Characteristics of steroid users in an adolescent school population. J Alcohol Drug Educ 1992;38(1):43–9.
[49] DuRant RH, Middleman AB, Faulkner AH, et al. Adolescent anabolic-steroid use, multiple drug use, and high school sports participation. Pediatr Exerc Sci 1997;9:150–8.
[50] Gas GL, Griffith EH, Cahill BR, et al. Prevalence of anabolic steroids use among Illinois high school students. J Athl Train 1994;29(3):216–22.

[51] Terney R, McLain LG. The use of anabolic steroids in high school students. Am J Dis Child 1990;144:99–103.

[52] Whitehead R, Chillag S, Elliot D. Anabolic steroid use among adolescents in a rural state. J Fam Pract 1992;35(4):401–5.

[53] Johnson MD, Jay MS, Shoup B, et al. Anabolic steroid use by male adolescents. Pediatrics 1989;83(6):921–4.

[54] Luetkemeier MJ, Bainbridge CN, Walker J, et al. Anabolic-androgenic steroids: prevalence, knowledge, and attitudes in junior and senior high school students. Journal of American Health Education 1995;26(1):4–9.

[55] Windsor R, Dumitru D. Prevalence of anabolic steroid use by male and female adolescents. Med Sci Sports Exerc 1989;21(5):494–7.

[56] Yesalis CE, Streit AL, Vicary JR, et al. Anabolic steroid use: indications of habituation among adolescents. J Drug Educ 1989;19(2):103–16.

[57] Taylor WN. Hormonal manipulation: a new era of monstrous athletes. Jefferson (NC): McFarland; 1985.

[58] Field AE, Austin SB, Camargo CA Jr, et al. Exposure to the mass media, body shape concerns, and the use of supplements to improve weight and shape among male and female adolescents. Pediatrics 2005;116:214–20.

[59] Jessor R. Risk behavior in adolescence: a psychosocial framework for understanding and action. J Adolesc Health 1991;12:597–605.

[60] Middleman AB, Faulkner AH, Woods ER, et al. High-risk behaviors among high school students in Massachusetts who use anabolic steroids. Pediatrics 1995;96(2):268–72.

[61] Rich JD, Dickinson BP, Feller A, et al. The infectious complications of anabolic-androgenic steroid injection. Int J Sports Med 1999;20:563–6.

[62] Melia P, Pipe A, Greenberg L. The use of anabolic-androgenic steroids by Canadian students. Clin J Sport Med 1996;6:9–14.

[63] Parkinson AB, Evans NA. Anabolic androgenic steroids: a survey of 500 users. Med Sci Sports Exerc 2006;38(4):644–51.

[64] Perry PJ, Lund BC, Deninger MJ. Anabolic steroid use in weightlifters and bodybuilders: an internet survey of drug utilization. Clin J Sport Med 2005;15(5):326–30.

[65] Freed DL, Banks AJ, Longson D, et al. Anabolic steroids in athletics: crossover double-blind trial on weightlifters. BMJ 1975;2:471–3.

[66] Sadler MA, Griffiths KA, McCredie RJ, et al. Androgenic anabolic steroids and arterial structure and function in male bodybuilders. J Am Coll Cardiol 2001;37:224–30.

[67] Ishak KG, Zimmerman HJ. Hepatotoxic effects of the anabolic/androgenic steroids. Semin Liver Dis 1987;7:230–6.

[68] Hartgens F, Kuipers H. Effects of androgenic-anabolic steroids in athletes. Sports Med 2004; 34:513–54.

[69] Cicardi M, Bergamaschini L, Tucci A, et al. Morphologic evaluation of the liver in hereditary angioedema patients on long-term treatment with androgen derivatives. J Allergy Clin Immunol 1983;72:294–8.

[70] Pecking A, Lejolly JM, Najean Y. Hepatic toxicity of androgen therapy in aplastic anemia. Nouv Rev Fr Hematol 1980;22:257–65.

[71] Hickson RC, Ball KL, Falduto MT. Adverse effects of anabolic steroids. Med Toxicol Adverse Drug Exp 1989;4:254–71.

[72] Socas L, Zumbado M, Perez-Luzardo O. Hepatocellular adenomas associated with androgenic-anabolic steroid abuse in bodybuilders: a report of two cases and a review of the literature. Br J Sports Med 2005;39:E27.

[73] Glazer G. Arthrogenic effects of anabolic steroids on serum lipid levels. Arch Intern Med 1991;151:1925–33.

[74] National Institute on Drug Abuse Research Report—Steroid Abuse and Addiction. National Institutes of Health Education Publication No. 00-3721. Bethesda (MD): National Institutes of Health; 2000.

[75] Hartgens F, Reitjens G, Keizer HA, et al. Effects of androgenic-anabolic steroids on apolipoproteins and lipoprotein (a). Br J Sports Med 2004;38:253–9.
[76] Sullivan ML, Martinez CM, Gennis P, et al. The cardiac toxicity of anabolic steroids. Prog Cardiovasc Dis 1998;41:1–15.
[77] McKillop G, Todd IC, Ballantine D. Increased left ventricular mass in a bodybuilder using anabolic steroids. Br J Sports Med 1986;20:151–2.
[78] Urhausen A, Holpes R, Kindermann W. One and two-dimensional echocardiography in bodybuilders using anabolic steroids. Eur J Appl Physiol 1989;58:633–40.
[79] Di Luigi L, Romanelli F, Lenzi A. Androgenic-anabolic steroids abuse in males. J Endocrinol Invest 2005;28(Suppl 3):81–4.
[80] Straus RH, Liggett MT, Lanese RR. Anabolic steroid use and perceived effects in ten weight-trained women athletes. JAMA 1985;253:2871–3.
[81] Miles JW, Grana WA, Egle D, et al. The effect of anabolic steroid use on the biomechanical and histologic properties of rat tendon. J Bone Joint Surg Am 1992;74:411–22.
[82] Rogol A, Yesalis C. Anabolic-androgenic steroids and the adolescent. Pediatr Ann 1992;21:175–88.
[83] Dickinson BP, Mylonakis E, Strong LL. Potential infections related to anabolic steroid injection in young adolescents. Pediatrics 1999;103(3):694.
[84] Pope HG Jr, Katz DL. Psychiatric and medical effects of anabolic-androgenic steroid use. Arch Gen Psychiatry 1994;51:375–82.
[85] Yesalis C, Kennedy N, Kopstein A, et al. Anabolic-androgenic steroid use in the United States. JAMA 1993;270:1217–21.
[86] Copeland J, Peters R, Dillon P. Anabolic-androgenic steroid use disorders among a sample of Australian competitive and recreational users. Drug Alcohol Depend 2000;60:91–6.
[87] Kashkin KB, Kleber HD. Hooked on hormones? An anabolic steroid addiction hypothesis. JAMA 1989;262:3166–70.
[88] Giannini AJ, Miller N, Kocjan DK. Treating steroid abuse: a psychiatric perspective. Clin Pediatr (Phila) 1991;30:538–42.
[89] Kutscher EC, Lund BC, Perry PJ. Anabolic steroids: a review for the clinician. Sports Med 2002;32(6):286–96.
[90] Yesalis C, Bahrke M, Kopstein A, et al. Incidence of anabolic steroid use: a discussion of methodological issues. In: Yesalis C, editor. Anabolic steroids in sport and exercise. 2nd edition. Champaign (IL): Human Kinetics Publishers; 2000. p. 74–106.
[91] Goldberg L, Elliot D, Clarke GN, et al. Effects of a multidimensional anabolic steroid prevention intervention: the Adolescents Training and Learning to Avoid Steroids (ATLAS) program. JAMA 1996;276:1555–62.
[92] Goldberg L, Bents R, Bosworth E, et al. Anabolic steroid education and adolescents: do scare tactics work? Pediatrics 1991;87:283–6.
[93] Metzl JD. Performance-enhancing drug use in the young athlete. Pediatr Ann 2002;31(1):27–32.
[94] Bernhardt DT, Gomez J, Johnson MD, et al. Strength training by children and adolescents. Pediatrics 2001;107:1470–2.
[95] Faigenbaum AD, Zaichowsky LD, Wescott WL, et al. The effects of a twice-a-week strength training program on children. Pediatr Exerc Sci 1993;5:339–46.

PEDIATRIC CLINICS
OF NORTH AMERICA

Pediatr Clin N Am 54 (2007) 787–796

Testosterone Precursors: Use and Abuse in Pediatric Athletes

Troy M. Smurawa, MD[a,b,]*, Joseph A. Congeni, MD[a,b]

[a]*Northeastern Ohio Universities College of Medicine,*
4209 State Route 44, PO Box 95, Rootstown, OH 44272, USA
[b]*Division of Sports Medicine, Children's Hospital Medical Center of Akron,*
One Perkins Square, Akron, OH 44308, USA

The popularity of dietary supplement use in the athletic population is widely increasing in an attempt to enhance athletic performance. Marketing and anecdotal evidence promote the use of these supplements as performance enhancers without sufficient scientific research and data to substantiate their performance-enhancing claims. Testosterone precursors, also called prohormones, are precursors in the endogenous production of testosterone. Androstenedione (Andro), dehydroepiandrosterone (DHEA), and androstenediol are the three testosterone precursors that are marketed heavily. The efficacy and safety of these prohormones were not well established, but they were believed to have the same androgenic effects on building muscle mass and strength as anabolic-androgenic steroids (AASs). The theory is to increase the body's endogenous production of testosterone by increasing the concentration of testosterone precursors exogenously. The short- and long-term side effects also were not well known, but theoretically they may cause the same adverse side effects as AASs.

In 1994, the Dietary Supplement Health and Education Act allowed for the marketing and sale of "natural" dietary supplements without the US Food and Drug Administration (FDA) regulation for guaranteeing the purity and safety of these substances. The passage of the Dietary Health and Education Act of 1994 allowed for theses precursors to be sold over the counter as "natural" dietary supplements without regulation.

In 1996, androstenedione and DHEA became available in the United States market as over-the-counter nutritional supplements. Dosages as high as

---

* Corresponding author. Division of Sports Medicine, Children's Hospital Medical Center of Akron, One Perkins Square, Akron, OH 44308.
E-mail address: tsmurawa@chmca.org (T.M. Smurawa).

0031-3955/07/$ - see front matter © 2007 Elsevier Inc. All rights reserved.
doi:10.1016/j.pcl.2007.05.002   *pediatric.theclinics.com*

androstenedione,100 to 300 mg per day, and DHEA,150 mg per day, were recommended [1]. These prohormones became an attractive performance-enhancing alternative to using illegal AASs, which were banned by most major sports organizations. They were classified as natural substances and were not regulated by the FDA. They became popular supplements among athletes, and, thus, became readily available to the adolescent population.

The potential performance-enhancing benefits of testosterone precursors were brought to the attention of the public and athletic community in 1998 when Major League Baseball player Mark McGwire set the home run record and openly admitted to using androstenedione [2]. Sales skyrocketed by 500%, and many supplements containing prohormones became available in the United States market. Questions and concerns of contamination with other supplements arose but their purity was unknown because these supplements were not regulated by the FDA. Also, their popularity was fueled by the misperception that nutritional supplements are natural, and, therefore, safe.

In 2004, after much controversy and debate, the US Department of Health and Human Services (HHS) and the FDA announced a crackdown on companies that manufacture, market, and distribute products containing androstenedione [3]. They recognized the potential serious adverse health risks that were similar to those associated with AASs. As part of their concern about its safety, the FDA and HHS sent warning letters to 23 companies asking them to stop distributing dietary supplements that contained androstenedione and warned them that enforcement actions would be taken if they did not comply. As a result of this action, the Anabolic Steroid Control Act of 2004 was passed. This act added the steroid precursor androstenedione to the list of schedule III controlled substances in the United States [4]. Schedule III substances have limited medicinal use, require a prescription from a licensed physician, and allegedly can threaten public health without government regulation. DHEA was not added to the controlled substance list; industry lobbyists contended that it had proven effective as an antiaging supplement and that its risks were minimal [4].

Use in pediatrics and adolescents

The extent of the use of testosterone precursors, such as androstenedione and DHEA, in the pediatric and adolescent population is unknown. The initial over-the-counter dietary supplement status and availability more than likely led to a large increase in the number of adolescents using testosterone precursors. A 2002 survey of 475 high school students by Reeder and colleagues [5] revealed that 4% of athletes and nonathletes admitted to using steroid precursors in the past year. Surveys by the National Collegiate Athletic Association (NCAA) revealed that 5.3% of athletes admitted to using DHEA or androstenedione, 33.4% admitted to using nutritional supplements, and 1.2% admitted to using anabolic steroids [6]. With the passage of the Anabolic Steroid Control Act of 2004, androstenedione became illegal to purchase; the only available source is through the black market or acquaintances. One would surmise that the use of testosterone precursors among adolescents would be higher than the use of AASs. Studies have found the rate of anabolic steroid use among junior and senior high students to be in the range of 3% to 7% [7–9]. This indicates that the trend for the use of performance-enhancing substances is no longer restricted to elite athletes but is pervasive in the pediatric and adolescent population. The lure of scholarships, product endorsements, and million-dollar salaries increases the pressure to get the competitive edge and the win-at-all-costs attitudes among young athletes.

Physiology

Testosterone precursors are involved in the endogenous production of testosterone. DHEA is produced naturally in the adrenal glands and gonads. DHEA is converted to androstenedione or androstenediol in the steroid synthesis pathway. Androstenedione and androstenediol are converted to testosterone in the testes and any tissue cells that contain androgen or estrogen receptors [10,11]. Adipose, bone, muscle, breast, prostate, liver, brain, and skin can be affected. The conversion of androstenedione and androstenediol to testosterone is regulated by the enzymes 17b-hydroxysteroid dehydrogenase and 3b-hydroxysteroid dehydrogenase, respectively.

The increased circulating levels of androstenedione and testosterone can be aromatized to estrone and estradiol [11–13]. Gonadal production of testosterone and estrogen is regulated by a negative-feedback system. The peripheral conversion of androgens and estrogens depends upon the quantity of circulating steroid precursors and not on any physiologic regulation system (Fig. 1) [12,14].

These precursors bind poorly to androgen receptors and have few inherent androgenic-anabolic properties. The theory is that by increasing the circulating concentration of steroid precursors, the body's endogenous production of testosterone increases and promotes anabolic effects in peripheral tissues [15,16]. It has been found that low to moderate doses of these precursors do not increase testosterone levels significantly; however, at high doses, testosterone levels can be increased significantly. Therefore, the increased testosterone levels may build muscle mass, increase strength, and improve athletic performance [15].

Efficacy in performance enhancement

Athletes use testosterone precursors with the belief that they will boost testosterone levels and, thereby, achieve the same anabolic effects of

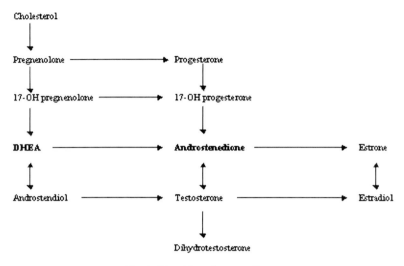

Fig. 1. Steroid syntheses pathway.

AASs. They are promoted to enhance performance by reducing fat, building muscle mass, increasing strength, and improving sexual performance. Studies of the efficacy of these testosterone precursors have not demonstrated any significant improvements in enhancing performance. The "Andro Project" by Broeder and colleagues [17] in 2000 studied the effects of healthy men, 35 to 65 years of age, taking androstenedione or androstenediol, 200 mg daily, in the setting of a 12-week high-intensity resistance-training program. Total testosterone levels increased by 16% after 1 month, but had returned to pretreatment levels by the end of the 12 weeks. The study also found that estrone and estradiol levels remained elevated significantly (up to 97%). Neither androstenedione nor androstenediol significantly improved lean body mass or increased muscle strength compared with placebo. They also found that there was an adverse effect on high-density lipoprotein (HDL) cholesterol and an increase in the coronary heart disease risk.

Brown and colleagues [18,19] studied the effects of daily oral supplementation with androstenedione, 300 mg, or DHEA, 150 mg, in healthy men 19 to 29 years of age with 8 weeks of resistance training. They found that serum androstenedione levels were elevated, but no significant increases in testosterone levels occurred, and it did not significantly enhance the adaptations to resistance training with changes in body composition or strength. They also examined the effects of a single dose of DHEA, 50 mg, and found a 150% increase in androstenedione levels within 60 minutes but no increases in testosterone levels.

A 2002 review of studies by Ziegenfuss and colleagues [1] found that most studies showed (1) acute oral ingestion of androstenedione or androstenediol, at least 200 mg, modestly and transiently increased serum testosterone levels in men; (2) elevation of circulating estrogen levels; (3) dosages of androstenedione or androstenediol, less than 300 mg/d for as long as 12 weeks, had no effects on body composition, muscle mass, or performance; and (4) significantly decreased serum HDL cholesterol levels and increases in the cardiovascular disease risk. A summary of research from 1999, which was published by Powers [16] in 2002, showed a consensus in that no significant increases in muscle mass or strength was found with a single dose or daily ingestion. High dosages of androstenedione, 200 to 300 mg/d, significantly increased serum testosterone levels in young healthy men by 34% and increased estradiol levels by 128%. The increases in testosterone levels were temporary, and daily doses up to 12 weeks showed significant increases in estradiol and estrone levels but did not show any significant increases in baseline testosterone levels. Other studies also showed no increase in muscle protein synthesis with supplementation with DHEA or androstenedione [20–22] and no increase in muscle fiber cross-sectional area with a combination of androstenedione ingestion and resistance training compared with placebo [21,23,24]. Studies also showed that androstenedione supplementation in men increased serum androstenedione levels; a low daily dose (100 mg) did not increase serum testosterone levels significantly, but a high daily dose (300 mg) increased serum testosterone levels and serum estrogen levels [17,20,23,25]. Investigations on the efficacy of DHEA, with dosages up to 150 mg/d, revealed no change in testosterone levels nor significant changes in lean muscle mass or strength compared with placebo [26–30].

Several reasons have been suggested for the lack of efficacy of androstenedione on improving muscle mass and strength. First, oral supplementation must undergo first-pass hepatic metabolism before it reaches the circulation. Second, only 2% of an oral dose is converted to testosterone; a large percentage is converted to testosterone glucuronide, which is biologically inactive. Third, the peripheral aromatization of testosterone to estradiol may limit the available level of testosterone to bind and activate androgen receptors [1,17,20,23,25].

In summary, the testosterone precursors DHEA, androstenedione, and androstenediol have little inherent androgen action. The ergogenic claims regarding prohormone supplementation have not been supported by controlled studies. Studies have demonstrated repeatedly that acute and long-term administration of oral androstenedione, androstenediol, or DHEA does not effectively increase serum testosterone levels and fails to produce any significant changes in lean body mass, muscle strength, or performance improvement compared with placebo. High doses of androstenedione seem to increase serum levels of estrogens, primarily through peripheral aromatization.

Safety and adverse effects

The adverse effects of oral supplementation with testosterone precursors are not well known. The lack of long-term studies makes it difficult to identify the dangers and risks of using these nutritional supplements. Adverse effects are most likely underreported because it is difficult to determine the prevalence of prohormone use and the disparity in product labeling of nutritional supplements. DHEA was reported to cause irreversible virilization in women (hair loss, hirsutism, deepened voice) and gynecomastia in men [31]. Androstenedione use was found to have an adverse effect on coronary heart disease risk and to cause a significant reduction in serum HDL cholesterol [20–22]. Long-term increased levels of unopposed circulating estrogens potentially could induce hormone-sensitive malignancies, such as uterine, breast, and prostate cancer [32]. Theoretically, high doses of prohormones could increase androgen levels and have the same adverse as AAS use, such as liver dysfunction, glucose intolerance/diabetes, malignancies, menstrual irregularities, infertility, testicular atrophy, impotence, male pattern baldness, acne, or aggressive behavior.

Studies are especially lacking in the pediatric and adolescent populations. Children and adolescents are vulnerable to the potential irreversible effects of androstenedione conversion to sex hormones. These effects could result in irreversible virilization in girls that is associated with hirsutism, severe acne, deepening of the voice, enlargement of the clitoris, menstrual irregularities, and even infertility. Excessive estrogens in boys can lead to feminization with testicular atrophy, impotence, and gynecomastia. Boys and girls potentially could experience precocious puberty, stunted growth, and premature closing of epiphyseal growth plates [23,28,29].

The public has the false perception that nutritional supplements are natural, and, therefore, safe. In fact, studies found that prohormone preparations often are contaminated with products that are not listed on the label, including AASs [33,34]. An International Olympic Committee (IOC)-funded study of 634 nonhormonal nutritional supplements found that 14.8% of these supplements contained prohormones that were not listed [35]. Baume and colleagues [36] analyzed the composition of 103 dietary supplements purchased on the Internet and found many contaminated with AASs. One out of five supplements was contaminated with chemicals not declared on the label, and creatine and mental enhancers were found to contain prohormones not listed on the label. Athletes and consumers need to be aware that the purity of nutritional supplements is not guaranteed; taking these supplements may result in a positive drug test and can subject the users to the adverse effects that are associated with AASs. As a result of increasing scientific evidence indicating real and significant health risks with the use of androstenedione products, the FDA and HHS initiated a campaign to educate consumers and cease the distribution, marketing, and sale of dietary supplements that contain androstenedione [37].

Legal issues

Several questions are raised when discussing the legal issues of a performance enhancing supplement. Is it safe? Does it work? Is it legal or fair? Most performance-enhancing supplements are not illegal but are banned by major sports-governing bodies. Testosterone precursors are banned by most major sports, including the IOC, National Football League, NCAA, Federation of International Football Association (FIFA), National Basketball Association, and Major League Baseball. As a result of the Anabolic Steroid Control Act of 2004, androstenedione is listed as a schedule III controlled substance and is regulated by the FDA [4]. DHEA was not placed on the controlled substance list. Theoretically, doping with androstenedione and DHEA can increase testosterone levels in the body, which increases levels of urinary testosterone secretion and can result in a positive urine drug test [33]. Also, many performance-enhancing supplements are contaminated with AASs and can result in a positive drug test [33,34]. Studies have demonstrated that the 7-Keto DHEA metabolites 7-hydroxylated-DHEA compounds are present endogenously in small amounts; however, these metabolites are abundant after the ingestion of exogenous 7-Keto DHEA [34,38]. The metabolites of 1-androstenediol androstenalone and 1-androstenedione are detectable for up to 120 hours after ingestion. Currently, only qualitative analysis is available, and doping analysis will require quantitative analysis and determination of appropriate threshold values. Further research and development of reliable drug tests will be needed to adequately test for doping with these agents.

Current medical recommendations

Current evidence shows that the testosterone precursors DHEA, androstenedione, and androstenediol do not offer any substantial performance-enhancing benefits. The potential adverse effects of these substances produce a significant health risk, especially to the pediatric and adolescent population. At higher doses, they were shown to minimally and temporarily elevate testosterone levels and to increase estrogen levels. No significant health or medical benefits exist, except for the possible antiaging properties of DHEA. As a result of the increasing evidence of the potential harmful health effects of these prohormones, the FDA has placed androstenedione on the schedule III controlled substance list and has not approved androstenedione or DHEA for any indication [4].

Summary

Dietary supplement use is increasing in the athletic population in an attempt to enhance athletic performance and gain a competitive edge.

Marketing and anecdotal evidence promote the use of these supplements as performance enhancers, often without sufficient scientific evidence to substantiate their performance-enhancing claims. Three testosterone precursors that have come on the market after the passing of the Dietary Supplement Health and Education Act of 1994 are androstenedione, DHEA, and androstenediol.

These testosterone precursors have little inherent androgen action. The ergogenic claims regarding prohormone supplementation have not been supported by controlled studies. Studies have demonstrated repeatedly that acute and long-term administration of oral androstenedione, androstenediol, or DHEA does not effectively increase serum testosterone levels and fails to produce any significant changes in lean body mass, muscle strength, or performance improvement compared with placebo. High doses of androstenedione seem to increase serum levels of estrogens, primarily through peripheral aromatization.

The extent of the use of testosterone precursors, such as androstenedione and DHEA, in the pediatric and adolescent population is unknown. It seems reasonable to believe that the use of testosterone precursors among adolescents is higher than the use of AASs. The adverse effects of oral supplementation with testosterone precursors are not well known. The lack of long-term studies makes it difficult to identify the dangers and risks of using these nutritional supplements. Consumers need to be aware that "natural" does not imply safety and the need to determine the efficacy, purity, safety, and legality of these supplements before using them is imperative. Studies are especially lacking in the pediatric and adolescent populations. Children and adolescents may be vulnerable to the potential irreversible effects of conversion to sex hormones.

Testosterone precursors are banned by most major sports, including the IOC, National Football League, NCAA, FIFA, National Basketball Association, and Major League Baseball. As a result of the Anabolic Steroid Control Act of 2004, androstenedione is listed as a schedule III controlled substance and is regulated by the FDA. Quantitative drug testing for doping needs to be well established to better monitor and control illicit use. No scientific data exist to support the medical use of these supplements. Health care professionals need to stay updated on current research and be well informed to discuss supplement use with individual athletes.

References

[1] Ziegenfuss TN, Berardi JM, Lowrey LM, et al. Effects of prohormone supplementation in humans: a review. Can J Appl Physiol 2002;27(6):628–45.
[2] Juhn MS. Popular sports supplements and ergogenic aids. Sports Med 2003;33:921–39.
[3] US Federal Drug Administration press release. HHS launches crackdown on products containing andro. Available at: www.cfsan.fda.gov/~;dms/andrlist. Accessed March 11, 2004.
[4] Denham BE. The Anabolic Steroid Control Act of 2004: a study of political economy of drug policy. J Health Soc Policy 2006;22(2):51–75.

[5] Reeder BM, Rai A, Patel DR, et al. The prevalence of nutritional use among high school students: a pilot study. Med Sci Sports Exerc 2002;34(Suppl 1):S1–62.
[6] NCAA. Study of substance use of college student athletes. 2006. Available at: www.ncaa.org/library/research/substance_use_habits/2006/2006_substance_use_report. Accessed March 14, 2007.
[7] Buckley WE, Yesalis CE, Friedl KE, et al. Estimated prevalence of anabolic steroid use among male high school seniors. JAMA 1998;260:3441–5.
[8] Yersalis CE, Barsukiewicz CK, Kopstein AN, et al. Trends in anabolic-androgenic steroid use among adolescents. Arch Pediatr Adolesc Med 1997;151:1107–205.
[9] Faigembaum A, Zaichowsky LD, Gardner DE, et al. Anabolic steroid use by male and female middle school students. Pediatrics 1998;1:e6.
[10] Earnest CP, Olson MA, Broaeder CE, et al. In vivo 4-androstene-3,17-dione and 4-androstene-3beta,17beta-diol supplementation in young men. Eur J Appl Physiol 2000;81:229–32.
[11] Labrie F, Luu-The V, Lin S, et al. The key role of 17beta-hydroxysteroid dehydrogenase in sex steroid biochemistry. Steroids 1997;62:148–58.
[12] Baulieu EE. Dehydroepiandrosterone (DHEA): a fountain of youth? J Clin Endocrinol Metab 1996;81:3147–51.
[13] Longcope C, Kato T, Horton R. Conversion of blood androgens to estrogens in normal adult men and women. J Clin Invest 1969;48:2191–201.
[14] Kretser DM, Risbridger GP, Kerr JB. Functional morphology. In: DeGroot LJ, Jameson JL, editors. Endocrinology. 4th edition. Philadelphia: WB Saunders; 1995. p. 2209–31.
[15] Abromowicz M. Creatine and androstenedione: two dietary supplements. Med Lett 1998;40:105–6.
[16] Powers ME. The safety and efficacy of anabolic steroid precursors: what is the scientific evidence? J Athl Train 2002;37(3):300–5.
[17] Broeder CE, Quindry J, Brittingham K, et al. The andro project. Arch Intern Med 2000;160:3093–104.
[18] Brown GA, Vukovich MD, Reifenrath TA, et al. Effects of anabolic precursors on serum testosterone concentrations and adaptations to resistance training in young men. Int J Sport Nutr Exerc Metab 2000;10(3):340–59.
[19] Brown GA, Vukovich MD, Sharp RL, et al. Effect of oral DHEA on serum testosterone and adaptations to resistance training in young men. J Appl Physiol 1999;87(6):2274–83.
[20] Rasmussen BB, Volpi E, Gore DC, et al. Androstenedione does not stimulate muscle protein anabolism in young healthy men. J Clin Endocrinol Metab 2000;85:55–9.
[21] Tokish JM, Kocher MS, Hawkins RJ. Ergogenic aids: a review of basic science, performance, side effects, and status in sports. Am J Sports Med 2004;32(6):1543–53.
[22] Wells S, Jozefowicz R, Statt M. Failure of dehydroepiandrosterone to influence energy and protein metabolism in humans. J Clin Endocrinol Metab 1990;71:1259–64.
[23] King DS, Sharp RL, Vukovich MD, et al. Effect of oral androstenedione on serum testosterone and adaptations to resistance training in young men: a randomized controlled trial. JAMA 1999;281:2020–8.
[24] Medical and nonmedical uses of anabolic-androgenic steroids: AMA Council on Scientific Affairs. JAMA 1990;264:2923–7.
[25] Brown GA, Vukovich MD, Martin ER, et al. Endocrine responses to chronic androstenedione intake in 30 to 50 year old men. J Clin Endocrinol Metab 2000;85(11):4074–80.
[26] Nissen SL, Sharp RL. Effects of dietary supplements on lean mass and strength gains with resistance exercise: a meta-analysis. J Appl Physiol 2003;94:651–9.
[27] Wallace BM, Lim J, Cutler A, et al. Effects of deyhdroepiandrosterone vs androstenedione supplementation in men. Med Sci Sports Exerc 1999;31(12):1788–92.
[28] Leder BZ, Longcope C, Catlin DH, et al. Oral androstenedione administration and serum testosterone concentration in young men. JAMA 2000;283(6):779–82.
[29] Leder BZ, Catlin DH, Longcope C, et al. Metabolism of orally administered androstenedione in young men. J Clin Endocrinol Metab 2001;86(8):3654–8.

[30] Nestler JE, Barlascini CO, Clore JN, et al. Dehydroepiandrosterone reduces serum low den-
     sity lipoprotein levels and body fat but does not alter insulin sensitivity in men. J Clin Endo-
     crinol Metab 1988;66:57–61.
[31] Congeni J, Miller S. Supplements and drugs used to enhance athletic performance. Pediatr
     Clin North Am 2002;49:435–61.
[32] Abromowicz M. Dehydroepiandrosterone (DHEA). Med Lett Drugs Ther 1996;38(985):
     91–2.
[33] Delbeke FT, Van Eonn P, Van Thuyne W, et al. Prohormones and sport. J Steroid Biochem
     Mol Biol 2002;83:245–51.
[34] Ayotte C, Levesque J, Cleroux M, et al. Sports nutritional supplements: quality and doping
     controls. Can J Appl Physiol 2001;26(Suppl):S120–9.
[35] International Olympic Committee. Analysis of nonhormonal nutritional supplements for
     anabolic-androgenic steroids. Available at: www.olympic.org http://multimedia.olympic.
     org/pdf/en_report_324.pdf. Accessed March 14, 2007.
[36] Baume N, Mahler N, Kamber M, et al. Research of stimulants and anabolic steroids in
     dietary supplements. Scand J Med Sci Sports 2006;16:41–8.
[37] FDA White Paper. Health effects of androstenedione. Available at: http://www.fda.gov/oc/
     whitepapers/andro.html. Accessed March 11, 2004.
[38] Lapcik O, Hampl R, Hill M, et al. Immunoassay of 7-hydroxysteroids: radioimmunoassay of
     7alpha-hydroxy-dehydroepiandrosterone. J Steroid Biochem Mol Biol 1999;71:231–7.

PEDIATRIC CLINICS

OF NORTH AMERICA

Pediatr Clin N Am 54 (2007) 797–806

Sports Medicine:
Performance-Enhancing Drugs

Andrew J.M. Gregory, MD, FAAP, FACSM[a,b,*],
Robert W. Fitch, MD[a,b]

[a]Vanderbilt University Medical Center, MCE–South Tower, Suite 3200, Nashville,
TN 37232, USA
[b]Vanderbilt University, MCE–South Tower, Suite 3200, Nashville, TN 37232, USA

Primary Care Sports Medicine has evolved as a field because of the need for physicians who are able to take care of the whole athlete and not just their orthopedic needs. This includes medical problems (eg, exercise-induced asthma or concussion), mental disorders (eg, eating disorders or anxiety), as well as an understanding of how medications affect training and exercise. To protect the athlete, physicians who take care of athletes need to be able to educate coaches, parents, and athletes about the benefits and risks of performance-enhancing drugs from a scientific perspective.

First, physicians must educate themselves regarding performance-enhancing drugs because this is not a subject taught in medical school or residency; however, we also must be cautioned not to contribute to the problem because, historically, many physicians have been the ones providing these drugs to the athletes (eg, steroids for Olympic programs in East Germany or blood doping in the Tour de France). Regardless, if we are employed by the team or acting voluntarily, the team physician must keep the best interests of the athlete above everything else.

Performance-enhancing drugs, ergogenic aids, or sports supplements have been a part of sports since sporting competition began and likely always will be. Considered cheating by purists and necessary by some athletes, we must accept the fact that they are used, understand why they are used, and study how to prevent their use to institute change. This article summarizes current scientific information regarding the use of

* Corresponding author. Vanderbilt Sports Medicine Center, MCE—South Tower, Suite 3200, Nashville, TN 37232.
E-mail address: andrew.gregory@vanderbilt.edu (A.J.M. Gregory).

performance-enhancing drugs in young athletes so that physicians can take the information and knowledgably educate others.

For this discussion, a drug refers to any substance that exerts an effect on a body system, and a supplement refers to a substance that is taken to augment the diet. Most vitamins and minerals are benign in nature and are difficult to misuse; however, some supplements (stimulants, steroid precursors) clearly are drugs and have the potential to cause significant morbidity and death. The categorization of these more significant substances with the more safe ones leads people to think that all supplements are safe; therefore, they are taken without consideration of harmful effects.

There are many different drugs and supplements used by athletes to enhance performance. Some of the more common classes are blood doping, anabolic steroids, stimulants, growth hormones, amino acids, and proteins [1]. Several of these products—although initially believed to be ineffective—have been shown to be good at increasing strength, decreasing fatigue, and building muscle. Although some of these products are illegal, they are readily available through prescription, supplements, local gyms, and the Internet (mostly from Mexico).

Because dietary supplements are treated differently than drugs by the US Government, supplement manufacturers do not have the same production standards as drug manufacturers. Supplement dilution or contamination is common as the same containers are used to process multiple different supplements without cleaning out the residue from the first. US Pharmacopeia and Consumer Labs perform purity testing and publish results on the different products from supplement manufacturers.

The US Food and Drug Administration (FDA) is responsible under the Federal Food, Drug, and Cosmetic (FD&C) Act for ensuring that manufacturers of foods, including dietary supplements, provide safe ingredients for their products as well as accurate, complete labeling that is truthful and not misleading [2]. Dietary supplements are treated as foods, as long as no drug claims are made for them. When products are marketed for therapeutic use, FDA regulates them through its Center for Drug Evaluation and Research.

The Nutrition Labeling and Education Act of 1990 (NLEA) [3], which amended the FD&C Act, provides the FDA with specific authority to require nutrition labeling of most foods and to require that all nutrient content claims and health claims be consistent with agency regulations. This drew the attention of supplement companies who were concerned that the FDA would now have additional authority over dietary supplements. They lobbied that the FDA would now be choosing for consumers what they could and could not have.

The Dietary Supplement Health and Education Act (DSHEA) of 1994 [4], which amended the NLEA, limits the FDA's authority by imposing a more relaxed standard for claims on supplements than for conventional foods. It defines a dietary supplement as a product intended to supplement the diet that contains one of the following ingredients: vitamin, mineral, herb or other botanical, amino acid or a concentrate, metabolite, constituent, extract, or combination of any ingredient. The Act shifts the burden of proof of safety from the manufacturer to the FDA. The Act also permits health claims if they accurately represent the current state of scientific evidence concerning the relationship between the supplement and a disease or other health-related condition, a determination that is left to the manufacturer.

Since the DSHEA of 1994, the FDA has proven several ingredients to be harmful and, therefore, required that they be removed from dietary supplements. Ephedra (ephedrine alkaloids) was the first to be banned in 2004 because of concerns over its cardiovascular effects, including increased blood pressure, irregular heart rhythms, and death. Also, in 2004, the Anabolic Steroid Control Act [5,6] was passed in the US Congress. It amends the Controlled Substances and Anabolic Steroids Control Acts to clarify the definition of anabolic steroids and to provide for research and education activities relating to steroids and steroid precursors. In addition to adding steroid precursors to the controlled substances list, it increased penalties for anabolic steroid offenses near sports facilities.

The most recent Act is the 2006 Dietary Supplement and Nonprescription Drug Consumer Protection Act, which mandates manufacturers of supplements and over-the-counter products to report serious adverse events to the FDA within 2 weeks of the claim. Manufacturer contact information is now required on the label, and all records of claims must be kept on file. It is hoped that these recent changes will protect the athletes from potential adverse events from products sold in supplements.

Although the Drug Enforcement Agency historically has concentrated on street drugs, in 2002 they began prosecuting manufacturers, distributors, and consumers of anabolic steroids. Victor Conte, who was the founder of BALCO Labs in San Francisco and the manufacturer of THG (tetrahydragestrinone), was arrested in 2004. Albert Saltiel-Cohen, a Mexico City veterinarian and owner of three of the largest steroid-manufacturing companies in the world, was arrested in 2005 in San Diego. In 2007, the owners of Signature Pharmacies in Orlando, Florida were arrested for fraudulently prescribing steroids and human growth hormone over the Internet.

Given the fact that young athletes use supplements and steroids, it behooves us to review what exactly they are using and why. There are few studies on side effects—especially long-term—and none at all in children. Most adolescent athletes do not make the most of their diet for performance before considering supplements. Most public high schools do not have drug-testing programs and are not likely to have them because of the cost. We are not sure that testing is an effective deterrent to use, but we do know that education works.

A 2003 survey showed that high school athletes frequently use supplements, including sports drinks, vitamin and minerals, energy drinks, herbal supplements, guarana, creatine, protein, and coenzyme Q10 [7]. They reported that they use them because of perceived short-term health benefits, prevention of illness, improved immunity, parental supply, taste, energy boost, better sports performance, and to rectify a poor diet.

In 15,000 adolescents from the 2006 National Longitudinal Study of Adolescent Health, boys were more likely than were girls to use anabolic steroids and legal supplements [8]. High school sports participation was associated with an increased likelihood that adolescents would use legal supplements in young adulthood. There was also a positive relationship between the use of legal dietary supplements and anabolic steroid use.

In a 2006 study of high school athletes in Nebraska, one quarter reported currently taking supplements [9]. Sports performance was the most reported reason for use, and their coach was listed as their best source of information on supplements. An anonymous survey of football and volleyball players from 20 high schools in northwest Iowa in 2001 showed that 8% of the male athletes and 2% of the female athletes were using supplements [10]. These included creatine, androstenedione, beta-hydroxy beta-methylbutyrate, amino acids, dehydroepiandrosterone, Phosphogen, Weight Gainer 1850, *Tribulus*, Muscle Plus, multivitamins, calcium, Gamma-aminobutyric acid, Shaklee Vita Lea, and Physique.

A survey of national track and field athletes competing at the 2004 World Junior Championships reported that 62% of respondents used supplements [11]. Of those, use among female athletes (75%) was higher than among male athletes (55%). Seventeen different supplements were reported, with an average of 2.5 products each (mostly multivitamins and minerals). Persons with the most influence on practices included coaches (65%), sports dieticians (30%), and doctors (25%).

In 1994, a questionnaire administered to all athletes at nine high schools in one rural county in Minnesota showed that 38% used supplements, equally by gender and grade in school [12]. Athletes with aspirations to participate in college sports were more likely to consume supplements. Healthy growth, treating illness, and sports performance were the most important reasons reported for supplement use. Parents, doctors, and coaches were reported as being the greatest influences on use. Most athletes believed that supplement consumption improved athletic performance. In 1995, the Nutritional Supplement Use and Knowledge Scale found that greater knowledge about supplements was associated with less use [13].

Protein supplements often are used by athletes with the hopes of adding muscle or repairing muscle damage from workouts. They are sold as powders to be used in shakes and taken directly before or after a workout. Most Americans consume the recommended daily allowance for protein each day. Unless the athlete is vegetarian and does not get protein from another source, supplementation is not indicated or necessary for building muscle. Although protein supplementation seems to be safe, if taken at the doses recommended, a significant protein load is placed on the kidneys. If this occurs during a period of dehydration, such as in a particularly intense workout in hot or humid conditions, the kidneys are at risk for acute failure.

Creatine probably is the protein supplement that is used most commonly by athletes for increasing strength [14]. It was discovered in the 1920s and made popular by Mark McGwire in Major League Baseball in the 1990s. It is a protein that is stored in skeletal muscle that binds phosphate to serve as an energy substrate for ATP. Creatine has demonstrated improved performance in repeated bouts of high-intensity strength work and sprints. There are no demonstrated effects in single-sprint activities, endurance exercise, or competition. Therefore, it is useful for increasing training intensity and volume to enhance physiologic adaptation.

One to 2 g of creatine per day are synthesized in the kidney, liver, and pancreas from the essential amino acids arginine, glycine, and methionine. An additional 1 to 2 g/d are obtained from a meat-containing diet. Once the muscle stores are saturated, the remaining creatine is converted to creatinine and cleared by the kidneys. Creatine is sold in a powder or liquid form in recommended dosages sometimes greater than 10 g/d. Taking dosages greater than 2 g/d is unnecessary and potentially harmful to the kidneys. There are two case reports of worsening renal failure in children who had underlying kidney disease using creatine. Other reported side effects include weight gain (water weight), nausea, and muscle cramping. Overall, creatine seems to be safe in adults, but no study has been performed specifically in children.

In 2000, students aged 14 to 18 years were surveyed regarding creatine during their preparticipation screen at a single institutional sports medicine center in Minnesota [15]; 8.2% of athletes reported creatine use, and half were taking creatine at the time of the survey. Most users believed creatine improved their performance and did not know how much creatine they were taking or were taking greater than the recommended dosage. They were more likely to know other creatine users and to use other supplements. Most obtained information from friends and purchased it from health food stores.

In 2001, athletes from 37 public high schools in Wisconsin took part in a cross-sectional, multisite, anonymous, descriptive survey of creatine use [16]; 16.7% of the athletes (25.3% boys, 3.9% girls) reported using creatine, from 8% in the 9th grade to 25% in the 12th grade. The sport with the lowest use was female cross country (1%), and football was the sport with the highest use (30%). For football, use differed by grade: 10.4% of grade 9 athletes and 50.5% of grade 12 athletes reported using creatine [17]. School size was inversely proportional to use, with 41% of players at small schools and 29% of players at large schools reporting use. Increased strength was the most likely perceived benefit, whereas dehydration was cited most often as a perceived risk. Users were encouraged to use most often by their friends, whereas their parents discouraged its use.

In 2001, 1103 middle and high school athletes aged 10 to 18 years in Westchester County, New York were surveyed before their preparticipation screen [18]. Six percent of athletes admitted taking creatine in all grades (6–12), but the highest use was found among the twelfth-grade students (44%). Use was higher in boys (9%) than in girls (2%) and was more common in football, wrestling, hockey, gymnastics, and lacrosse. Users reported enhanced performance and improved appearance as the most common reasons for use. Safety was cited as the most common reason for not using.

Androgenic-anabolic steroids (AASs) are perhaps the best known and most widely publicized of the performance-enhancing drugs. Shown to be effective by the East German Olympic athletes in the 1950s, steroids are known to permeate the sports of weight lifting, body building, professional wrestling, and the Olympics. Anabolic steroids include derivatives and precursors of the hormone testosterone. Testosterone exerts many effects on the body, including increasing protein synthesis and euphoria and decreasing catabolism. Initially, the medical community demonstrated that steroids were not effective, but the tests were conducted using physiologic dosing instead of what the athletes were using (10–100 times that).

There is no doubt now that steroids work; however, the potential side effects are significant and must be taught to athletes. These include decreased testosterone production, testicular atrophy, and gynecomastia in boys and masculinization in girls. Cardiovascular effects are substantial, with clotting, myocardial infarction, stroke, and death topping the list. If the injectable form is used, aside from disease transmission risks, hepatitis, cholestasis, and even, carcinoma can form in the liver. Psychologic effects are common, including aggression, dependence, anxiety, depression, and psychosis. In adolescents, early epiphyseal closure and increased suicidal ideation and attempts have been described. Mood swings and irritability may be clues to anabolic steroid use as well as drug abuse.

A 2000 systematic review showed that adolescent anabolic steroid users were significantly more likely to be boys and to use other illicit drugs, alcohol, and tobacco. It also showed that student athletes were more likely than were nonathletes to use steroids. Football players, wrestlers, weightlifters, and bodybuilders had significantly higher prevalence rates.

In 2002, the Project EAT: Eating Among Teens study was performed on 4746 middle and high school students from St. Paul/Minneapolis public schools. They completed surveys and anthropometric measurements regarding eating patterns and weight concerns. Reported steroid use was 5.4% in boys versus 2.9% in girls. In boys, AAS use was associated with poorer self-esteem, depressed mood, attempted suicide, poorer knowledge and attitudes about health, greater participation in sports that emphasize weight and shape, greater parental concern about weight, disordered eating, and substance use. Among girls, steroid use was less consistent in its associations with other variables.

In 1999, varsity football players in Indiana were selected randomly from 27 high schools to complete a questionnaire. Out of 873 subjects, 6.3% were current or former AAS users. The average age at time of first use was 14 years, but 15% began taking before the age of 10 years. Half of the respondents indicated that they could obtain AASs if they so desired. Other athletes, physicians, and coaches were listed as sources for AASs.

In 1998, a confidential self-report questionnaire was administered to male and female students, 9 to 13 years of age, from four public middle schools in Massachusetts. The response rate was 82% (965/1175 eligible), and 2.7% of all middle school students reported using steroids (boys and girls). More steroid users than nonusers believed that steroids make muscles bigger and stronger, improve athletic performance, make one look better, were not bad for them, knew someone their own age who currently took steroids, were asked by someone to take steroids, and reported that they would take steroids in the future.

In 2006, 2924 Norwegian high school students (age 15–19 years) were surveyed at 5-year intervals; 1.9% reported the use of AASs in 1994 and 0.8% reported their use in 1999. By multivariate logistic regression, future AAS use was predicted by young age, male gender, previous AAS use, power sports participation, and frequent alcohol use.

The 1997 Centers for Disease Control and Prevention Youth Risk Behavior Surveillance was a nationally representative sample of more than 16,000 United States public and private high school students; 6.1% of students in high school had taken illegal anabolic steroids. Binge drinking, cocaine use, fighting, and sexual risk-taking were associated with higher odds of lifetime steroid use. Neither athletic participation nor strength conditioning predicted the odds of steroid use after controlling for problem behaviors. Steroid-using athletes reported the same frequency of use as did steroid-using nonathletes.

Stimulants may be the most widely and underrecognized supplement used by high school athletes and yet are the least studied. Common stimulants include caffeine (guarana [*Paullinea cupana*]), ephedrine (ephedra or ma huang), pseudoephedrine, Neo-Synephrine, amphetamines, and methamphetamines. Stimulants can be found in coffee, colas, energy drinks, cough and cold medications, muscle building or weight loss supplements, attention-deficit/hyperactivity disorder (ADHD) medication, and diet pills. Most studies on stimulant use are with medication used to treat ADHD and not on use with athletics. There are a few studies on their use for athletic performance in adults, but no studies have been done in the young.

Stimulants act on the central nervous system (CNS) to increase arousal, respiratory rate, heart rate, and blood pressure and, therefore, improve performance. Side effects can include dizziness, insomnia, agitation and restlessness, anxiety, confusion, paranoia, hallucinations, dyskinesias, gastrointestinal disturbances, heat intolerance, stroke, myocardial infarction, arrhythmia, and death. Severe rebound of fatigue and depression occurs after discontinuance. Contraindications for stimulant use include heart disease, strokes, high blood pressure, thyroid disease, diabetes, or seizures.

Drug testing has drawn a lot of attention recently for use in high schools because several states have mandated it (eg, New Jersey, Texas). There is a long history of drug testing at the Olympic level, which is now centralized through the World Anti-Doping Agency. Testing is now required in most professional sports, the National Collegiate Athletic Association (NCAA), and most colleges and universities. Testing is difficult, expensive, and always lags behind what athletes are currently using. Until it is known what substance is being used, a test cannot be created to find it and sometimes one may never be available (ie, autologous blood). There is no solid evidence that drug testing prevents use, except when the athletes know that a test is imminent; however, many states are considering steroid testing in public high schools.

In 2006, Aegis Labs in Nashville, Tennessee did drug tests for more than 60 high schools. From the approximately 30 private and 30 public high school accounts, they tested more than 3000 samples. Fifty-six schools tested for drugs only, 3 schools tested for steroids and drugs, and 7 schools tested for steroids only. There are multiple testing profiles—none of which is all-inclusive—but each costs less than $100.

Of the high school samples tested, 543 were positive (16.6% of the total) for drugs of abuse. By far, the most positives were for CNS stimulants (116 amphetamine, 36 pseudoephedrine, 34 cocaine [benzoylecgonine, a metabolite], 3 methylenedioxymethamphetamine [Ecstasy], 1 phentermine, 1 methamphetamine), followed by CNS depressants ([opioids: 14 morphine, 13 hydrocodone, 6 oxycodone, 3 codeine], alcohol [17 ethyl alcohol], and barbiturates [1 phenobarbital, 1 butalbital]), hallucinogens (marijuana metabolite - 37 carboxy-tetrahydrocannabinol), and, finally, antianxiety drugs (6 alprazolam) (Dr. David Black, personal communication, 2007).

We do drug testing at our institution as a means of monitoring for athletes who may need help with substance abuse and preventing positive tests at the NCAA level. The samples are collected by the certified athletic trainer randomly and for cause. After a positive result we require weekly counseling regarding drug and alcohol use as well as weekly testing until deemed no longer necessary by the counselor. There are no penalties for the first offense, a 1-year suspension for the second offense, and disqualification from athletics for the third offense.

Although drug testing has not been proven to prevent drug abuse, education of athletes by coaches, parents, and allied health professionals has proven to be beneficial in prevention. In a 2002 study, 40 high school students from a low-income community were separated into experimental and control groups [19]. The experimental group was given five lessons on various nutrition and sport supplement topics. Both groups were administered a validated nutrition and sport supplement questionnaire consisting of 28 questions before and after. Postintervention scores improved 9 points in the experimental group, from 6 to 15, but did not change in the control group.

A 2004 Swedish health promotion program intervention targeted all 16- and 17-year-old boys and girls to create awareness of, and to discuss attitudes toward, steroid hormones among these adolescents. Youth leaders and health workers discussed these subjects with adolescents over a period of 2 years. The intervention was well received by the adolescents, and the misuse of AASs had a tendency to decrease after the program.

Two drug prevention programs were designed specifically for high school athletes by Oregon Health & Science University. The ATLAS (Athletes Training and Learning to Avoid Steroids) drug prevention program is directed at male athletes and the ATHENA (Athletes Targeting Healthy Exercise & Nutrition Alternatives) is for female athletes. ATLAS is a hands-on approach with interactive activities. It uses coaches and peer leaders as facilitators in a team setting. There are 10 45-minute interactive classroom sessions and three exercise sessions regarding sports nutrition, exercise alternatives, the effects of substance abuse in sports, drug refusal role-playing, and the creation of health promotion messages. The goal is to reduce risk factors that foster the use of anabolic steroids and other drugs by using the athletic team to deter drug use and promote healthy nutrition and exercise as alternatives.

The second program, ATHENA is a school-based, team-centered prevention program for female athletes on sports, dance, and cheer teams. It consists of eight 45-minute sessions integrated into their usual sport-training activities. It is designed to reduce disordered eating and the use of diet pills and other supplements, as well as promote healthy nutrition and exercise. This program has not been proven to prevent eating disorders.

Further information regarding the ATLAS or ATHENA programs can be obtained through the Oregon Health & Science University at 503/494-3727, kolmers@ohsu.edu, or by visiting the Web site (www.atlasprogram.com). The price of the 4- to 5-hour training program is charged per participant (minimum of 20 and maximum of 100) plus travel expenses and program materials.

The ATLAS program was tested in 31 high school football teams that consisted of 3207 athletes in three successive annual cohorts (1994–1996) [20]. Intentions to use and actual AAS use were significantly lower among participants. Although actual AAS reduction was not significant at 1 year, intentions to use AASs remained lower and students used less sport supplements and had improved nutritional behaviors.

We know that many young athletes use drugs for sports enhancement and that most are not aware of the potential risks of their use. Education of athletes works for the prevention of supplement and steroid use. As physicians who take care of young athletes, we need to be the ones to educate coaches and parents, who, in turn, will educate their athletes. We also have opportunities to discuss this with athletes during preparticipation screening or office visits for other sports-related complaints. Testing likely will always be too expensive and impractical to be used effectively at the high school level. We also need to work with the FDA to clarify dietary supplements from drugs so that we can protect consumers against potential adverse events.

References

[1] Johnson RJ, et al. Current review of sports medicine. 2nd edition. Philadelphia: Current Medicine Inc.; 1998.
[2] Farley Dixie. Dietary supplements: making sure hype doesn't overwhelm science. FDA Consumer Magazine 1993.

[3] Guide to Nutrition Labeling and Education Act (NLEA) Requirements; August 1994.
[4] Dietary Supplement Health and Education Act of 1994; Public Law 103–417.
[5] Anabolic Steroids Control Act of 1990; Public Law 101–647.
[6] Anabolic Steroid Control Act of 2004–Amendment to the Controlled Substances Act; 108th CONGRESS; 2d Session; S. 2195; March 2004.
[7] O'Dea JA. Consumption of nutritional supplements among adolescents: usage and perceived benefits. Health Educ Res 2003;18(1):98–107.
[8] Dodge TL, Jaccard JJ. The effect of high school sports participation on the use of performance-enhancing substances in young adulthood. J Adolesc Health 2006;39(3):367–73.
[9] Scofield DE, Unruh S. Dietary supplement use among adolescent athletes in central Nebraska and their sources of information. J Strength Cond Res 2006;20(2):452–5.
[10] Mason MA, Giza M, Clayton L, et al. Use of nutritional supplements by high school football and volleyball players. Iowa Orthop J 2001;21:43–8.
[11] Nieper A. Nutritional supplement practices in UK junior national track and field athletes. Br J Sports Med 2005;39(9):645–9.
[12] Sobal J, Marquart LF. Vitamin/mineral supplement use among high school athletes. Adolescence 1994;29(116):835–43.
[13] Massad SJ, Shier NW, Koceja DM, et al. High school athletes and nutritional supplements: a study of knowledge and use. Int J Sport Nutr 1995;5(3):232–45.
[14] Kraemer WJ, Volek JS. Creatine supplementation. Its role in human performance. Med Sci Sports Exerc 1999;31(8):1147–56.
[15] Smith J, Dahm DL. Creatine use among a select population of high school athletes. Mayo Clin Proc 2000;75(12):1257–63.
[16] McGuine TA, Sullivan JC, Bernhardt DA. Creatine supplementation in Wisconsin high school athletes. WMJ 2002;101(2):25–30.
[17] McGuine TA, Sullivan JC, Bernhardt DT. Creatine supplementation in high school football players. Clin J Sport Med 2001;11(4):247–53.
[18] Metzl JD, Small E, Levine SR, et al. Creatine use among young athletes. Pediatrics 2001;108(2):421–5.
[19] Little JC, Perry DR, Volpe SL. Effect of nutrition supplement education on knowledge among high school students from a low-income community. J Community Health 2002;27(6):433–50.
[20] Goldberg L, MacKinnon DP, Elliot DL, et al. The adolescents training and learning to avoid steroids program: preventing drug use and promoting health behaviors. Arch Pediatr Adolesc Med 2000;154(4):332–8.

ELSEVIER
SAUNDERS

PEDIATRIC CLINICS

OF NORTH AMERICA

Pediatr Clin N Am 54 (2007) 807–822

Gene Doping: A Review of Performance-Enhancing Genetics

Gary R. Gaffney, MD[a],*, Robin Parisotto, BA[b]

[a]*Division of Children and Adolescent Psychiatry, Department of Psychiatry, University of Iowa College of Medicine, 200 Hawkins Road, Iowa City, IA 52242, USA*
[b]*International Centre for East African Running Science, Glasgow University, Glasgow, Scotland*

The World Anti-Doping Agency (WADA) [1] defines gene doping as "the non-therapeutic use of genes, genetic elements and/or cells that have the capacity to enhance athletic performance." The WADA Code is the ethical document developed by the quasi-governmental organization, in partnership with the International Olympic Committee, to pioneer and coordinate sports antidoping efforts around the world. Without a single known human incident of gene doping, WADA bestowed the technique of gene doping a dishonored place on the list of prohibited substances.

For an entire biomedical technique to be banned, before even acquiring regulatory approval by any government or before acceptance by any branch of organized medicine, seems to be unprecedented [2]. Why would a sports regulatory administration express such preemptive concern about a putative medical technique of the future? This article answers that question and predicts the future of gene doping.

Drug doping uses therapeutic advances in exercise physiology and clinical pharmacology to provide unfair advantages to athletes who covertly use anabolic drugs, thus dramatically enhancing competitive performance. Similar to drug doping, gene doping manipulates scientific advances originally developed for the treatment of disease. Rather than drug interventions, the gene-doping athletes appropriate advances in gene therapies. Gene doping, in concept, uses scientific developments that manipulate DNA in the most basic regulation of biologic processes, to dramatically improve aspects of athletic performance, such as speed, power, or endurance [2–10].

Molecular biology, particularly the "discovery" of DNA by Watson and Crick in 1953, revolutionized biology and medicine. The rate of genetic

---

* Corresponding author.
E-mail address: gary-gaffney@uiowa.edu (G.R. Gaffney).

0031-3955/07/$ - see front matter © 2007 Elsevier Inc. All rights reserved.
doi:10.1016/j.pcl.2007.04.004   *pediatric.theclinics.com*

discovery in molecular biology rapidly accelerated throughout the last half of the twentieth century and into the twenty-first century. The new millennium was to be the dawning of practical, effective treatments for genetic diseases, such as muscular dystrophy, X-linked hemophilia, and other single-gene disorders [5]. Further, with molecular biology advances that included insertions of new genes into organisms, cloning of organisms, and use of human stem cells, more than single-gene diseases could be treated. Any number of serious or fatal medical conditions might be altered with the introduction of genes that would produce "in vivo pharmacies" delivering biochemicals, including proteins and hormones, to injured or impaired tissue.

Gene therapy also could improve a general disadvantageous condition, such as aging-related muscle atrophy, by introducing a transgene to produce the depleted factors involved in muscle repair and regeneration [5]. Therapeutic genes could be targeted directly into cells, tissues, and organs limiting effects to a localized site, thus reducing the systemic side effects produced by a typical drug administration.

Implications of novel genetic interventions fascinated not only researchers, physicians, and gene therapists, but also coaches, athletes, and trainers looking for athletic performance enhancement of biologic parameters, such as strength, power, and oxygen delivery, to create a critical edge in sporting competition [5]. The creation of a superman or superwoman athlete could be planned by well-placed genetic physiologic tweaks.

Background: from performance-enhancing drugs to performance-enhancing genes

Drug cheats in sports long used steroid hormones, amphetamines, and blood manipulations to achieve advantages in competition (performance-enhancing drugs or PEDs [9]. Steroid hormones produced rapid gains in muscle size, strength, and recovery. Amphetamines improved alertness and concentration. Blood doping improved oxygen delivery to tissues allowing more endurance in competition; however, each of these drugs/manipulations showed significant side effects. Steroids produced atrophy of sex organs, gynecomastia, emotional rages, and other serious side effects. Amphetamines reduced appetite and—in large doses—produced paranoid or psychotic symptoms. Blood doping resulted in a hematocrit so high that the erythrocytosis caused thrombosis and embolism. These blood dyscrasias, combined with erythropoietin (EPO)-related serious cardiac effects, seemed to be particularly lethal [9].

As laboratory detection become more sophisticated in catching drug cheats, the athletes turned to novel peptides, such as human growth hormone (HGH), to gain an edge or to avoid detection by antidoping authorities. Substances like HGH were expensive and dangerous, however; HGH was harvested from cadavers, some of whom died from contagious spongiform neurologic conditions. Other peptide hormones, including EPO, which regulates red blood cell (RBC) production, remained unavailable as drugs.

The emerging biotechnology industry changed these limitations with the implementation of recombination DNA production of peptide drugs and hormones. Manipulating genes inserted into mammalian cells, the new industry produced recombinant (r) drugs, such as rHGH, rEPO, insulin-like growth factor (r-IGF)-1, and r-insulin in great quantities. Essentially identical to human hormones, these advanced drugs produced a significant impact on the medical treatment of anemia, growth deficiency, and diabetes, for example; however, biotechnology advances did not go unnoticed by the coaches and athletes who look for every advantage in competition [5].

Soon after introduction of a new recombinant peptide or hormone, the sports doping community appropriated the drug if it offered an advantage in competition. Unscrupulous physicians and trainers used rHGH and rIGF-1 to increase strength and power among a wide variety of athletes, including Major League Baseball and National Football League players. rEPO proliferated among cycling competitors to increase oxygen delivery to muscles during lengthy and demanding races like the Tour de France.

The detection of these new recombinant DNA–produced peptide hormones in rogue athletes presented formidable challenges that continue to be problematic for antidoping laboratories [9,10]. Although the use of rHGH, rEPO, and insulin in sports like football, cycling, track, and baseball is widespread, antidoping laboratories continuously must play catch-up in developing detection procedures. Thus, the introduction of recombinant drugs into the sports doping field might be considered the first step in genetic-related doping.

With the advent of gene therapy, a more direct way to deliver proteins and hormones to an athlete's tissues and organs became reality. The sophistication and the power of these biologic alterations piqued the ingenuity of the drug-cheating coaches and athletes. A substance that can alter the basic genetic expression of DNA—such that muscles grow larger, contract more forcefully, and recover more quickly than non-doped muscles—and cannot be detected by antidoping laboratories would be ideal to gain a competitive advantage while not running afoul of the regulatory officials.

Genetic therapies

In the broad sense, genetic therapies include several categories of biotechniques [7,9,10]:

1. Use of recombinant DNA techniques to produce new peptides or drugs (rEPO)
2. Pharmacogenetics, or the use of knowledge of the specific genome of an athlete to tailor pharmacologic interventions

3. Somatic cell modification, which produces genetically modified cells (eg, modified RBCs to increase blood-carrying capacity)
4. Germ-line modification, where the gametes or early embryos undergo gene modification to express more athletically expedient traits
5. Genetic preselection, where a gene scan would inform parents about the distribution of desired genes in a potential offspring
6. Genetic selection, where individuals are selected for particular traits (widely practiced in animal husbandry)

This article's main focus is on the modification of cells to express proteins or other biochemicals to enhance athletic performance.

Defined as "the transfer of genetic material to human cells for the treatment or prevention of a disease or disorder," gene therapy uses genetic materials, such as DNA, RNA, or genetically altered cells [3]. In the simplest form, gene therapy introduces a "therapeutic gene" (transgene) into an organism by way of a vector, often an inactive virus. Within the organism itself, the new "transgene" synthesizes the defective/missing protein or biologic substance to correct dysfunctional tissues and organs. Other gene therapy strategies involve manipulation of genes, turning them on or off as the desired physiologic response dictates.

Initial gene therapy trials included protocols to treat an X-linked immunodeficiency disease and hemophilia variant [5]. A trial of human vascular endothelial growth factor produced positive results in patients who had angina [10]. More than 1000 gene therapy trials are ongoing in various states of clinical study [2,6,7]. No gene therapy protocols have been approved for medical practice by the US Food and Drug Administration, the regulatory agency charged with overseeing the development and clinical use of the medical procedure.

Genetic enhancement

Gene doping also could use the technique of genetic enhancement/engineering. In practice in agricultural settings, genetic enhancement places advantageous genes into organisms, not to cure disease, but to confer advantages to the organism that would improve the organism's survival or the organism's "product": hardiness, better insect resistance, or greater yield. Genetic enhancement exploits the same techniques as gene therapy; however, it can be applied outside of medicine [3].

Genetic performance enhancement: gene doping

Using basic principles of gene therapy (and genetic enhancement), gene doping injects genes directly into the athlete's body by one of two methods: in vitro delivery and ex vitro delivery [5,10]. In gene therapy, the clinician introduces a gene that covers for a deficient gene or modulates the activity of an existent gene to correct a disease state. The goals of gene doping include the injection of novel genes or the modulation of existing genes too; however, the gene doper introduces the gene products for the enhancement of physiologic parameters expedient to the athlete's competitive tasks, rather than the treatment of a medical illness.

In vivo gene doping

The delivery of the new gene into the athlete can be through biologic, physical, or chemical methods. Viruses can be modified to biologically insert the artificial gene into cells in a specific organ or target tissue or into cells throughout the competitor's body. Virus lines modified to transfer genes to mammalian cells include retroviruses, adenoviruses, and lentiviruses [10,11]. Physical methods to deliver genes into cells use microsyringes, or gene guns. Biochemical injection vehicles use plasmids or liposomes [10,11].

Ex vivo gene doping

The technique of exogenous gene doping involves gene transfer to cells in culture first, then implantation of the tissue into the recipient. Once implanted into the athlete's cells, the new genes express hormones or biochemicals that again enhance tasks of the athlete in competition [11].

Candidate genes for athletic gene doping

Any physiologic process involved in producing a motor action or assisting in the implementation of a motor movement could be a candidate for gene doping (Table 1; Fig. 1). The physiologic processes of pulmonary respiration, cardiovascular circulation, oxygen delivery, striated muscle growth/efficiency/repair, and even neuromuscular coordination could be altered to give an athlete an edge over his or her competition. Although more esoteric, neurophysiologic processes, such as mental alertness, motivation, and central nervous system recovery, also might be amenable to gene doping. The list of physiologic processes related to athletic competition is long and likely only limited by current understanding of exercise physiology and exercise psychology [10].

Even now, in the exploratory phase of gene therapy/gene doping, there are obvious candidates for the aspiring gene cheat. These primary gene candidates exist as targets of biomedical researchers looking for legitimate disease treatments [10].

Hematopoietic/vascular systems

The classic example of a genetic alteration to enhance athletic performance occurred naturally in 1964. A Finnish skier, Eero Mantyranta, dominated Olympic Nordic skiing. Studies later demonstrated that Mantyranta benefited

Table 1
Candidate genes for sports doping

Gene/product	System/organ targets	Gene product properties	Physiologic response
ACE	Skeletal muscles	Peptidyl dipeptidase	ACE-D is involved in fast twitch muscles ACE-I seems to correlate with endurance
ACTN3	Skeletal muscle	Actin-binding proteins related to dystrophin	Involved in fast twitch muscles
Endorphins	Central and peripheral nervous systems	Widely active peptides	Pain modulation
EPO	Hematopoietic system	Glycoprotein hormone	Increases RBC mass and oxygen delivery
HGH	Endocrine system	191–amino acid protein	Increases muscle size, power, and recovery
HIF	Hematologic and immune systems	Multisubunit protein	Regulates transcription at hypoxia response elements
IGF-1	Endocrine/metabolic/skeletal muscle	70–amino acid protein	Increases muscle size, power, and recovery by increasing regulator cells
Myostatin	Skeletal muscle	2-subunit protein	Regulates skeletal muscle. Inhibition increases muscle size, power, and recovery.
PPAR-delta	Skeletal muscle and adipose tissue	Nuclear hormone receptor protein	Promotes fat metabolism and increases number of slow twitch fibers
VEGF	Vascular endothelium	Glycosylated disulfide-bonded homodimers	Induces development of new blood vessels

Abbreviations: ACE, angiotensin-converting enzyme; ACTN3, actinin binding protein 3; EPO, erythropoetin; HGH, human growth factor; HIF, hypoxia inducible factor; IGF-1, insulin-like growth factor; PPAR-delta, peroxisome proliferators-activated receptor (delta); VEGF, vascular endothelial growth factor.

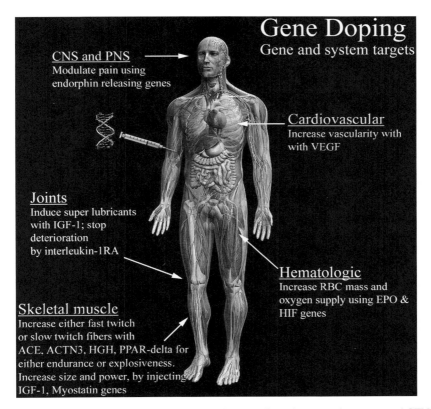

Fig. 1. Gene doping: gene and system targets. ACE, angiotensin converting enzyme; ACTN, actinin binding proteins; EPO, erythropoietin; HGH, human growth hormone; HIF, hypoxia inducible factor; IGF-I, insulin-like growth factor; PPAR-delta, peroxisome proliferator-activated receptor; VEGF, vascular endothelial growth factor.

from a natural mutation in the EPO gene that produced a greater number of RBCs, with a concomitant increased oxygen-carrying capacity [3,5]. This skier possessed what every blood doper in history tried to achieve—a physiologic advantage in delivering more oxygen to various tissues, including muscles.

rEPO (epoetin and darbopoetin) is a much-abused injected recombinant protein that increases RBC production, leading to increased oxygen-carrying capacity and oxygen delivery to tissues. The abuse of rEPO is epidemic in cycling, leading to frequent controversy, tedious forensic investigations, and serious side effects, including death [9].

Using gene doping, an additional EPO gene could be delivered to the athlete by way of a viral vector. Once in the athlete, the gene would express much more EPO than normally produced, even with training. The desired result would be an increase in the oxygen-carrying capacity of the blood, thus bestowing a clear competitive advantage in endurance sports.

Laboratory experiments have been successful in injecting the gene into monkeys and mice. Although the procedures successfully raised hematocrit, severe side effects, including a paradoxical anemia, resulted [12–15].

Hypoxia inducible factors

The hypoxia inducible factor (HIF) family of proteins modulates the activity of genes in low-oxygen environments. Various HIFs increase production of RBC, as well as increase cellular energy use. Enhancement of these proteins clearly would benefit the aerobic athlete [16–18].

Vascular endothelial growth factor

Clinical studies are currently ongoing for vascular endothelial growth factor (VEGF), a gene product that encourages development of new blood vessels [3]. This genetic manipulation would be advantageous to patients suffering from coronary artery disease. The gene-doping athlete would benefit from a putative increase in vasculature and more delivery of oxygen and nutrients to the peripheral tissues.

Skeletal muscle system

Actin-binding peptides

The proteins actin and myosin form the machinery of muscle contraction. The family of actin-binding proteins in humans includes α-actinin alleles ACTN2 and ACTN3. Alpha-actinins maintain the structure of the myofibrillar array and regulate myofiber contraction. A defect of ACTN3 regulation occurs when the ACTN3 gene codes for a premature stop codon; ACTN2 seems to compensate in these persons. Correlation studies found evidence that the ACTN2 endows muscular endurance traits upon athletes. Conversely, elite sprinters benefit from more copies of ACTN3. Depending on the event of the competitor, gene doping with the appropriate ACTN allele could enhance endurance capacity or sprint effectiveness [18].

Angiotensin-converting enzyme

Physicians are well aware of angiotensin-converting enzyme (ACE) inhibitors used for the treatment of hypertension; however, the ACE gene, like the ACTN gene, codes for proteins that seem to endow different exercise capacities. Research suggests that the ACE-I allele endows advantages in endurance, which would be useful for distance runners. The ACE-D allele seems to be associated with elite sprinting performance [18–20]. Again, a gene-doping athlete could inject the appropriate gene to influence better performance in his or her event, be it a sport featuring short bursts of speed and power or a sport in which endurance is the key to success.

Insulin-like growth factor

Several sophisticated studies, most notably at the University of Pennsylvania [5,21], targeted IGF-1, a peptide, in conjunction with HGH, intimately involved with muscle growth, repair, and power. These studies demonstrated eloquent ways in which IGF-1 controlled mammalian muscle development and demonstrated that targeted gene therapy could successfully produce hypertrophied and powerful muscles in laboratory mice. The primary investigator, Lee Sweeney, designed the procedure carefully so that the virus and the gene were not expressed systemically; by avoiding systemic distribution of the peptide, the researchers hoped to avoid the serious side effects of IGF-1, including myocardial hypertrophy and carcinogenesis. Thus, for therapeutic reasons, the researchers designed the gene therapy to be effective locally, in injected muscles. That particular feature also would benefit a doping athlete, because the transgene IGF-1 would not enter the systemic circulation where it might be detected by laboratory testing. In this University of Pennsylvania protocol, "fingerprints" of the gene therapy did occur; however, the theoretic aim of the study itself would present problems for antidoping agencies.

Myostatin

Myostatin, known to be a negative regulator of muscle development, presents another candidate gene. This regulator protein seems to turn-off muscle growth. Substances that block myostatin or genes that produce ineffective myostatin proteins would allow superphysiologic muscle growth in terms of number and thickness of cells (as seen in certain breeds of cattle through a natural mutation) [22,23]. Not only do striated muscles hypertrophy without myostatin regulation, but less fat is gained on the body of the animal. The manipulation of this regulatory protein has obvious advantages for the athlete.

Peroxisome proliferator-activated receptor delta

The peroxisome proliferator-activated receptor delta (PPAR-delta) gene seems to be a prime candidate for gene doping [24–26]. This gene codes for an increase in mitochondrial biogenesis and promotes an adapted muscle fiber transformation. The gene promotes an increase in type 1 muscle fibers (slow twitch). Elite athletes show an increase in PPAR-delta gene levels. A PPAR-delta gene was inserted into mice; it dramatically improved the animal's endurance capacity. It was concluded that "...these genetically generated fibers confer resistance to obesity with improved metabolic profiles, even in the absence of exercise. These results demonstrate that complex physiologic properties such as fatigue, endurance, and running capacity can be molecularly analyzed and manipulated."

Central and peripheral nervous system

Endorphins

In injuries, as well as in competition, pain limits athletic achievement. Athletes sustain countless painful injuries for which they consume an abundance of anti-inflammatory drugs and pain-relieving medicines. Likewise, the buildup of lactic acid during competition induces pain. Clearly, increasing the pain threshold—and alleviating the discomfort of nagging injuries—would improve performance.

The introduction of genes producing analgesic endorphins and enkephalins would increase the pain threshold in an athlete, for pain experienced in competition as a result of lactic acid buildup and pain due to acute and chronic injury. Clinical trials are testing the efficacy of genes encoding these natural narcotic peptides for pain relief in humans [3].

Other potential candidate genes

Interleukin-15 may prove to be an anabolic protein amenable to gene doping [27]. Interleukin-1RA gene injection trials reported good results; this gene could be used therapeutically for osteoarthritis and to promote joint superlubrication [28]. Mechano-growth factor may aid in the repair of damaged skeletal muscle tissue [9].

Risks and complications of gene doping

Examining the history of clinical pharmacology reveals that side effects of novel treatments can be unexpected and occasionally fatal. From thalidomide to valdecoxib, newly introduced medications, even with exhaustive preclinical trials, produce unanticipated untoward side effects. Consider the potential side effects of introducing a foreign gene, by way of a viral vector, into an organism's chromosomes. Gene therapy trials made headlines several times with unexpected and fatal side effects. Then 18, Jesse Gelsinger died in 1999 as the victim of an immune response to the virus used in a well-publicized gene therapy trial [4]. That death shocked the biomedical world and resulted in regulation as well as multiple legal actions. Several patients who were treated for an X-linked hemophilia with a gene therapy protocol developed leukemia, an obviously unexpected side effect [4].

A gene therapy trial of EPO in macaque monkeys produced such stimulation of RBC production that the monkeys' blood thrombosed [13]. Moreover, many of the monkeys suffered anemia, the result of an immune response to the gene therapy. The overactive immune response attacked endogenous EPO as well as gene-stimulated EPO [14]. A similar experiment using gene-therapy EPO revealed that the gene-induced EPO was slightly different from natural monkey EPO [15]. Likewise, the use of transgene

EPO in human gene doping might induce erythrocytosis to a dangerous level, with potentially lethal consequences.

Although not generally considered a risk from gene therapy, the virus vector could infect other humans. Clinical trials monitor subjects for viral shedding [3]. It would be unlikely that gene cheats would monitor their secretions for viral contamination. Furthermore, rogue gene-doping laboratories (like their steroid-synthesizing counterparts) would not implement proper preclinical trials. Thus, there may be a possibility of a modified infectious virus passing from a gene cheat to other persons.

If the experience with anabolic steroids is any indicator, athletes generally ignore common dosing recommendations. When a Maryland physician introduced the anabolic steroid methandrostenolone (D-bol) to power lifters in the 1960s, it was not long before the athletes increased the dose and the duration of drug beyond medical recommendations. Contemporary anabolic drug users stack multiple anabolic steroids mixed with other anabolic drugs in megadoses that lead to serious side effects and even death. A prominent and successful athlete like Barry Bonds, in a quest to become a more powerful hitter, allegedly used multiple anabolic substances including anabolic steroids, HGH, modafinil, insulin, clomiphene, and EPO [29]. Given this phenomenon with drug doping, expect the use of multiple gene-doping protocols by the athlete looking for every edge in competition. Genes for strength, power, recovery, analgesia, oxygen delivery, concentration, injury, and repair could be transferred to the same athlete. As with anabolic steroids and other PEDs, there will be unpredictable side effects and fatal interactions.

Laboratory detection of gene doping

Frequent battles occur between drug cheats, antidoping agencies, and the lawyers representing all sides. The drug cheats eternally search for an undetectable PED; thus, the antidoping laboratories play "catch-up" forensic detective in developing sensitive tests for any new PEDs. Elite sport has entered the world of forensics, where winners and losers of competitive events can be declared in the courtroom, not the playing field. Further, legal proceedings take months. Because of forensic procedures, the 2006 Tour de France will not declare a winner until months after the finish of the race. Are regulatory agency antidoping laboratories developing methods to detect possible gene-doping use, and will these methods stand up in court?

The WADA initiated research to prepare for the world of gene doping [2,4]. Research scientists suggest several biologic/laboratory tests that could operate to expose gene-doping cheats [2–4,9,10]. The usual parameters of laboratory tests—sensitivity, specificity, validity, and reliability—would need documentation to allow such innovative tests to withstand the certain legal scrutiny when elite athletes test positive for gene cheating.

Muscle biopsy

A biopsy of suspected muscle tissue could reveal viral vehicles or evidence of altered genes; however, that possibility presents a invasive and low-yield antidoping measure [2,4].

Blood monitoring

Proteins and hormones produced by doped genes could be exactly like endogenous proteins. Thus, it may be extremely difficult to detect the difference between the endogenous gene product and the doped-gene product; however, serial monitoring of blood parameters may reveal suspicious elevations of key biologic substances that indicate gene doping [2]. For instance, the dramatic increase in hematocrit, in conjunction with several other hematological parameters, could tip off a regulatory agency that an athlete used a gene-doping technique to improve oxygen delivery to muscles.

Genetic activity tests

Interesting developments could use patterns of gene activity or gene products to detect abnormal gene activity [2]. Detection of these patterns uses cutting-edge microchip gene array technology or nanotechnology breakthroughs. The monitoring or visualization of gene activity or gene products through the expression of DNA and RNA by a sophisticated microchip array could monitor thousands of genes, enabling the laboratory to use a sophisticated detective tool for gene doping [9].

Protein fingerprints

In this process, similar to gene microarray testing, hundreds of biologic proteins could produce a "protein fingerprint" or a "genetic map" of the biochemistry of individual athletes [10]. Suspicious alterations of such an individualized fingerprint or map would alert sporting authorities to possible gene doping.

Genetic barcodes

It may be possible to label the transgene products with a genetic "bar code"; however, this tactic would require the cooperation of a broad array of professionals from the research scientists to the pharmaceutical houses to the administrating physicians [4].

Regulation of gene doping

WADA is the preeminent doping regulatory agency in the world, concerning itself with the ethical application of medical techniques, therapies, and treatments in the realm of competitive sport. WADA develops the "code" and the "prohibited list" of banned substances for Olympic sport athletes [1–3,6,8].

The ethical criteria for a drug or medical technique to be included on the WADA prohibited list are "scientific evidence, proven pharmacological effect or experience that substances or methods included have the potential to enhance or enhances sport performance" [1–3,6,8]. Two arguments are used for inclusion on the list: the substance or method may be harmful or cause a health risk to the athlete and the use of doping violates the spirit of sport, as defined by WADA criteria. Essentially, the substance or technique is outside "fair play," which could be construed as "cheating."

The WADA tenets have been criticized as ambiguous [3]. Clearly, any medical intervention can be a health risk; athletic competition itself is a health risk. The key factor in determining the ethical use of a drug in athletic competitions rests on the point of fair play. When is a drug not given or taken for a therapeutic purpose, but for a purpose of obtaining an unfair competitive advantage? That ethical battle continues every day in many sporting venues. With the advent of gene therapy, the focus of the debate will turn from drugs to transgene products; however, the key element of therapeutic versus manipulative will remain unchanged.

Relevance of gene doping to the practicing pediatrician

Adolescent athletes use anabolic drugs. Studies estimate that approximately 2% to 4% of adolescents have used some sort of anabolic drug [30] by the time they graduate from high school. The entire story is not told, however, because most survey studies focus on anabolic steroids. Many teenage athletes possess sophisticated knowledge about anabolic drugs, such that use of HGH, insulin, and even EPO could appear in this age group. Sources of information about anabolic substances include the daily reports of the athletes suspected or caught using PEDs, peers at the local gym, and, occasionally, unethical coaches or trainers. Physicians must be alert for the use of PEDs in the at-risk age group and alert for side effects, including endocrine, behavioral, hematologic, and cardiovascular complications, of PED use [31].

If gene doping becomes reality among elite athletes, it is almost certain that adolescent athletes will be exposed to the technique. Either through their own volition or through peers, unscrupulous coaches, and overzealous parents, adolescents will try to gain a competitive advantage for the glory of athletic achievement and the scholarships that follow. Although the use of anabolic drugs and techniques increases once the athlete engages in college or professional sports, teenagers will use performance enhancing genetics (PEGs) when such techniques arrive in the gym. Thus, if the technique proves successful in elite athletes, gene doping will appear in the teenage population; pediatricians should prepare themselves for new syndromes and unusual side effects. A physician should understand the possible target organs and putative doping genes.

Although most clinical research and clinical reports concern athletes looking for a competitive advantage, nonathletes use anabolic substances for an enhancement of physical appearance. Exhibiting muscle dysmorphia or the Adonis Complex [32,33], these youth mimic the good looks and enhanced bodies of actors and models. A thriving black market delivers anabolic drugs to this group of adolescents for narcissistic purposes. If available, and if successful, expect teenagers to use gene-doping techniques for cosmetic purposes.

Perhaps the most sinister example of gene doping, in the broad sense, would be germ cell modification and genetic preselection [34]. In germ cell modification, a gamete or embryo would have DNA modified to enhance the expression of athletic advantageous genes. This technique, as futuristic as it sounds, would alter the entire genomic makeup of the developing human to produce a superior athlete.

In genetic preselection, the genome would be scanned, allowing parents to choose the most genetically athletically gifted offspring to survive. This process is a sophisticated twenty-first century variant of the ancient Spartan child-selection process. Although no reports exist of parents scanning the genome of their prospective children, there are reports of a sporting organization using a limited genome scan to select prospective athletes or to genetically tailor training [35].

Summary

Examination of the history of sports competition reveals unethical athletes who use medical advances, mostly pharmaceutics, to gain an edge in competition. The elucidation of the genetic basis of biology leaves medical science on the precipice of clinically useful gene therapy; however, it is expected that unscrupulous athletes and their mentors will divert the new techniques to gain an edge over competitors. Much remains to be determined in this area; however, a multitude of candidate genes exists [36]. The biologic techniques to introduce these genes into athletes are developing rapidly; it seems to be only a matter of time before the genetically enhanced performance athlete takes the field of competition. Sporting regulatory agencies initiate and maintain programs to monitor and test for gene doping. Physicians will be part of the professional net involved with these futuristic gene-enhanced athletes.

Although gene doping sounds like a science fiction plot, the physician should not underestimate the capacity of humans to find an edge in competition—legal or illegal. As athletes, professionals, parents, and coaches, the authors have experienced numerous examples of cheating in sports. From the simple falsification of player records to the importation of foreign athletes to the use of anabolic steroids and PEDs, athletes, coaches, boosters, parents, and physicians will bend the rules of fair play. The greater the stakes, the higher the rewards; the temptation to cheat becomes more alluring. If gene therapy becomes reality in humans—and the technique is poised to become clinically useful—those participants who hold no moral compunctions against cheating fellow competitors will use the technique. Indeed, officials expressed great concern that an unscrupulous coach was experimenting with gene doping at the 2004 Turin Olympics [37]. At some point in time, performance-enhancing genetics will be a reality; as professionals, be forewarned and be prepared.

Acknowledgments

The authors acknowledge Elizabeth Gaffney, Kyle Gaffney, and Willem Koert for their help in preparing the manuscript.

References

[1] World Anti-Doping Agency. The 2007 prohibited list: international standard. Montreal (Canada): WADA; 2006.

[2] Pincock S. Feature: gene doping. Lancet 2005;366(Suppl 1):S18–9.

[3] Haisma HL, de Hon O, Sollie P, et al. Gene doping. The Netherlands: Netherlands Centre for Doping Affairs; 2004.

[4] McCrory P. Super athletes or gene cheats? Br J Sports Med 2003;37:192–3.

[5] Sweeney HL. Gene doping. Sci Am 2004;291:62–9.

[6] Unal M, Unal DO. Gene doping in sports. Sports Med 2004;34(6):357–62.

[7] Trent RJ, Alexander IE. Gene therapy in sport. Br J Sports Med 2005;40:4–5.

[8] World Anti-Doping Agency. Gene doping. Play true, official publication of the World Anti-Doping Agency 2005;(1):2–6.

[9] Parisotto R. Blood sports: the inside dope on drugs in sport. Prahran (Victoria): Hardie Grant Books; 2006.

[10] Azzazy HME, Mansour MMH, Christenson RH. Doping in the recombinant era: strategies and counterstrategies. Clin Biochem 2005;38(11):959–65.

[11] Sinn PL, Sauter SL, McCray PB Jr. Gene therapy progress and prospects: development of improved lentiviral and retroviral vectors—design, biosafety, and production. Gene Ther 2005;12:1089–98.

[12] Svensson EC, Black HB, Dugger DL, et al. Long-term erythropoietin expression in rodents and non-human primates following intramuscular injection of replication-defective adeno-viral vector. Hum Gene Ther 1997;8(15):1797–806.

[13] Zhou S, Murphy JE, Escobedo JA, et al. Adeno-associated virus-mediated delivery of erythropoietin leads to sustained elevation of hematocrit in nonhuman primates. Gene Ther 1998;5(5):665–70.

[14] Goa G, Lebherz C, Weiner DJ, et al. Erythropoietin gene therapy leads to autoimmune anemia in macaques. Blood 2004;103(9):3300–2.

[15] Lasne F, Martin L, de Ceaurriz J, et al. "Genetic doping" with erythropoietin cDNA in primate muscle is detectable. Mol Ther 2004;10(3):409–10.

[16] Lippi G, Guidi GC. Gene manipulation and improvement of athletic performance: new strategies in blood doping. Br J Sports Med 2004;38:641.

[17] Zarember KA, Malech HL. HIF-1α: a master regulator of innate host defense. J Clin Invest 2005;155:1702–4.

[18] MacArthur DG, North KN. Genes and human elite performance. Hum Genet 2005;116(5): 331–9.

[19] Dekany M, Harbula I, Berkes I, et al. The role of insertion allele of angiotensin converting enzyme gene in higher endurance efficiency and some aspects of pathophysiological and drug effects. Curr Med Chem 2006;13(18):2119–26.

[20] Pitsiladis YP, Scott R. Essay: the makings of the perfect athlete. Lancet 2005;366(Supl 1): S16–7.

[21] Lee S, Barton ER, Sweeney HL, et al. Viral expression of insulin-like growth factor-1 enhances muscle hypertrophy in resistance trained rats. J Appl Physiol 2004;96(3):1097–104.

[22] Bogdanovich S, Krag TO, Barton ER, et al. Functional improvement of dystrophic muscle by myostatin blockade. Nature 2002;420(6914):418–21.

[23] Schuelke M, Wagner KR, Stolz LE, et al. Myostatin mutation associated with gross muscle hypertrophy in a child. N Engl J Med 2004;350(26):2682–8.

[24] Kramer DK, Ahlsen M, Norrbom J, et al. Human skeletal muscle fibre type variations correlate with PPAR α, PPAR δ and PGC-1 α mRNA. Acta Physiol (Oxf) 2007;189(1): 207–16.

[25] Grimaldi PA. Regulatory role of peroxisome proliferators-activated receptor delta (PPARδ) in muscle metabolism: a new target for metabolic syndrome treatment? Biochimie 2005; 87(1):5–8.

[26] Wang YX, Zhang CL, Yu RT, et al. Regulation of muscle fiber type and running endurance by PPAR-δ. PLoS Biol 2004;2:e294.

[27] Busquets S, Figueras M, Almendro V, et al. Interleukin-15 increases glucose uptake in skeletal muscle. An antidiabetogenic effect of the cytokine. Biochim Biophys Acta 2006; 1760(11):1613–7.

[28] Evans CH, Gouze JN, Gouze E, et al. Osteoarthritis gene therapy. Gene Therapy 2004;11: 379–89.

[29] Fainaru-Wada M, Williams L. Game of shadows. New York: Gotham Books; 2006. p. 271–5.

[30] Johnston LD, O'Malley PM, Bachman JG. Monitoring the future national results on adolescent drug use: overview of key findings, 2005. NIH Publication No. 06–5882. Washington, DC: National Institutes of Health; 2006.

[31] Calfee R, Fadale P. Popular ergogenic drugs and supplements in young athletes. Pediatrics 2006;117:577–89.

[32] Pope HG Jr, Gruber AJ, Mangweth B, et al. Body image perception among men in three countries. Am J Psychiatry 2000;157(8):1297–301.

[33] Choi PYL, Pope HG, Olivardia R. Muscle dysmorphia: a new syndrome in weightlifters. Br J Sports Med 2002;36:375–7.

[34] Gene Doping for beginners. Staun J. Playthegame. 2006. Available at: http://www.playthe game.org/Home/Knowledge%20Bank/Authors/Jakob%20Staun.aspx. Accessed February 25, 2007.

[35] Pincock S. Gene doping at Torino? The scientist. 2007. Available at: http://www.the-scien tist.com/news/display/23101. Accessed February 25, 2007.

[36] Rankinen T, Perusse L, Rauramaa R, et al. The human gene map for performance and health-related fitness phenotypes: the 2003 update. Med Sci in Sports Exerc 2004;36(9): 1451–69.

[37] Dennis C. Rugby team converts to give gene tests a try. Nature 2005;434:260.

Abuse of Growth Hormone Among Young Athletes

Sergio R.R. Buzzini, MD, MPH

Departments of Pediatrics and Orthopaedics, Geisinger Medical Center,
100 North Academy Avenue, Danville, PA 17822, USA

Professional sports figures have received significant media attention associated with allegations of abuse of growth hormone (GH) [1–11]. Many athletes and bodybuilders believe that GH improves athletic performance and appearance; however, scientific evidence suggests that, in healthy individuals, GH supplementation does not offer any advantage. Although only a few studies have investigated the abuse of GH among young athletes, the use of ergogenic substances by famous athletes has long encouraged young athletes and nonathletes to try them.

The existence of a growth-promoting factor from bovine anterior pituitary was discovered in 1921 [12]; however, it was first used as a treatment for dwarfism in 1932 [13]. Human GH (hGH) was isolated in 1944 [14]. The first purified preparation of hGH dates to 1956, and it was extracted from human cadaver pituitaries [15]. The first clinical use of hGH was reported in 1958 as a treatment for children who have GH deficiency (GHD) to promote linear growth [16]. Cadaveric supplies remained the only source of hGH for almost 3 decades. As a result, hGH was not widely available, and world demand far exceeded supply. The clinical use of hGH lasted until 1985, when its use was halted worldwide because of its association with Creutzfeldt-Jakob disease [17]. Since 1985, all GH in clinical use has been obtained by recombinant DNA technology through genetic engineering and is named recombinant hGH (rhGH). The use of this technology eliminated supply as the limiting factor [18,19]. Although GH has a number of accepted medical uses in the United States, GH also is widely used illegally as an antiaging agent and as a performance-enhancing substance in athletics. Published evidence does not indicate the use of GH as an antiaging treatment for healthy older adults [20]. Athletes and bodybuilders claim that GH has anabolic properties, increasing lean body

E-mail address: srbuzzini@geisinger.edu

0031-3955/07/$ - see front matter © 2007 Elsevier Inc. All rights reserved.
doi:10.1016/j.pcl.2007.07.002

mass and decreasing fat mass [21]. In 1989, the International Olympic Committee made GH a banned substance as part of a new doping class of "peptide hormones and analogues" [22], despite the lack of a legitimate test for GH.

The performance-enhancing potential of GH use in sports was first advocated in the *Underground Steroid Handbook* in 1983 [23]. Although it is believed that the use of GH is widespread in sports, evidence about its abuse is largely anecdotal and circumstantial because of the technical laboratory difficulties in detecting its abuse. After Ben Johnson was stripped of his 100-m gold medal from the Seoul Olympic Games in 1988, he admitted to having taken a cocktail of drugs containing rhGH [9]. It is believed that GH has become so popular with athletes that the 1996 Atlanta Olympics were known informally as the "Growth Hormone Games" [8]. At the 1998 Tour de France, a large number of vials of rhGH were detected in the possession of cycling teams [11]. A Chinese swimmer, Yuan Yuan was forced to withdraw from the 1998 World Championship in Perth, Australia after 13 vials of rhGH were discovered in her suitcase at the Sydney airport [1]. At the 2000 Olympic Games in Sydney, a coach from Uzbekistan was caught with a supply of rhGH [7], and a few months before the start of the games, 1575 vials of rhGH were stolen selectively from a pharmacy in Australia [3]. The sprinter Tim Montgomery (former 100-m world record holder) admitted using rhGH in 2001 [5], and New York Yankees slugger Jason Giambi admitted to injecting himself in 2003 with GH [6]. A physician prescribed rhGH to several players on the Carolina Panthers football team during the team's 2003 championship season [10]. In 2006, investigators for the US Government intercepted a package of rhGH sent to Arizona Diamondbacks pitcher Jason Grimsley [4]. More recently, the actor Sylvester Stallone was formally convicted of importing 48 vials of rhGH to Australia [2]. The use of GH is not limited to professional sports figures; 3.5% of college student-athletes reported using GH in the past 12 months [24], and 5% of male American high school students used or have used GH as an anabolic agent [25].

Growth hormone physiology

The human genome carries two genes encoding for GH [26]. The normal GH gene is transcribed and translated predominantly in the somatotrophs of the anterior pituitary gland [27]. The variant gene is transcribed in the placenta [28] and progressively replaces the pituitary GH in the circulation of pregnant women [29,30]. In addition, synthesis of GH occurs at several extrapituitary sites, including discrete neuronal populations within the central nervous system, epithelial cells of the mammary gland, endothelial cells of blood vessel fibroblasts, thymic epithelial cells, and cells of the immune system, including macrophages, B cells, T cells, and natural killer cells [31,32].

In circulation, hGH is present in multiple molecular isoforms and frag-
ments differing in size, binding affinities, immunoreactivity, and bioactivity
[33–35]. The predominant form is made up of 191 amino acids, has a molecular weight of 22 kd, and accounts for about 50% of all GH molecules.
The 20-kd monomer, which is devoid of amino acids 32 to 46, has 176
amino acids and accounts for about 10% of GH molecules. Other types
of GH include modified GH (30%), acidic GH (7%), and variable amounts
of fragmented GH [36,37]. The rhGH molecule is identical to the 22-kd
isoform.

The secretion of pituitary GH is regulated by two hypothalamic peptides:
GH-releasing hormone (GHRH), which stimulates GH secretion, and so-
matotropin release inhibiting hormone (SRIH), formerly called somatostatin,
which inhibits GH secretion [38]. Ghrelin, another peptide synthesized mainly
in the gastrointestinal tract in response to the availability of nutrients, also
stimulates GH secretion [39]. It is believed that ghrelin acts as a GHRH
through hypothalamic mechanisms [40]. Negative feedback occurs at two
levels: GH itself and insulin-like growth factor (IGF)-I reduce GH release
by the somatotropes through enhancing SRIH tone and reducing GHRH release. The continuous secretion of placental GH into maternal circulation during pregnancy is not affected by GHRH or SRIH [29,30].

The pituitary gland secretes GH in a pulsatile pattern that is modified by
gender and age [41–43]. In women, secretion of GH is higher, with lower
peaks and higher troughs [44,45]. Higher concentrations of GH are present
in neonates, and the highest levels are observed at puberty [46]. At puberty,
increasing levels of sex steroids alter the negative feedback effects and, therefore, increase levels of GH and IGF-I. Shortly after peak height velocity, secretion of GH decreases by around 14% per decade [47]. Moreover, GH
also is reduced in obesity [48], carbohydrate-rich diets, and the intake of
β2 adrenergic agonists. Conversely, GH secretion is higher during slow
wave sleep, exercise, hypoglycemia, amino acid intake (leucine and arginine), increased temperature, and stress [38]. Drugs, such as clonidine,
L-dopa, and γ-hydroxybutyrate, increase its secretions, as do androgens
and estrogens. After secretion by the pituitary gland, nearly 50% of circulating GH binds to a GH-binding protein (GHBP) [49,50]. This protein, produced by cleavage of the GH receptor (GHR), represents its extracellular
component [51,52]. Circulating GHBP might reflect the amount of GHR expressed [53]. GHR is composed of preformed dimers that undergo conforma-
tional change when occupied by a GH ligand, promoting signaling [54]. In
fact, the stoichiometry of 1:2 (hormone/receptor ratio) occurs as a consequence of two binding sites (GH sites 1 and 2) [55]. Depending on growth
hormone concentration and binding affinities of site 1 and 2, GH may exhibit
distinct effects ranging from full agonism to antagonism [56–58].

GHRs are present in all tissues in the body and stimulate many metabolic
processes. One of the best-known actions of GH is the generation of IGF-I
and its IGF-binding proteins (IGFBPs) [59] that prolong the half-life of

IGF-I in circulation. Among the IGFBPs, IGFBP-3 seems to be unique in having the capacity to bind a second ligand, ie, acid labile subunit; therefore, a three-component etero-trimeric complex is present in the circulation [60]. In most tissues, IGF-I has local autocrine and paracrine actions, but the liver is the main organ that secretes IGF-I (and IGFBPs) into circulation [61]. The actions of IGF-I include stimulation of cell proliferation and apoptosis inhibition [62]. In muscle, IGF-I affects protein synthesis by enhancing amino acid uptake and accelerating transcription and translation [63]. Although IGF-I levels usually reflect the integrated secretory activity of GH, IGF-I levels are regulated by other factors as well [64]. In fact, subtly elevated GH levels may not uniformly induce high IGF-I levels [65,66]. Therefore, circulating IGF-I should be considered more as a marker of GH action on the liver rather than the "second messenger" of GH action. In fact, the hypothesis of separate and distinct actions of GH and IGF-I on protein turnover has been suggested [67]. Levels of IGF-I are highest during late adolescence and decline throughout adulthood [68]; these levels are determined by gender and genetic factors [69] and are elevated during pregnancy. The production of IGF-I is suppressed in malnourished patients, such as in anorexia nervosa, as well as in patients who have liver disease, hypothyroidism, or poorly controlled type 1 diabetes.

Growth hormone pharmacodynamics

The serum half-life of free GH is about 20 minutes after secretion or intravenous injection [70,71] and is prolonged to several hours by binding to GHBP. After subcutaneous or intramuscular administration, blood concentrations of GH reach a peak between 1 and 3 hours after injection and decrease to undetectable levels after 24 hours [72]. Healthy adults secrete approximately 0.4 mg/d (18.6 nmol/d) and young adolescents secrete approximately 0.7 mg/d (32.5 nmol/d) of GH in circulation. In adults aged 30 to 50 years, endogenous GH production is approximately 0.2 mg/d in women and 0.1 mg/d in men [73]. When GH is measured in healthy persons with the use of standard assays, the level is usually undetectable (<0.2 µg/L throughout most of the day), but there are approximately 10 intermittent pulses of GH per 24 hours, most often at night, when the level can be as high as 30 µg/L [74]. In patients who have acromegaly, the endogenous secretion of GH often is increased more than 100-fold. The circulating GH is cleared from the bloodstream through degradation, predominantly in the liver and kidney [75]. Only minute quantities of GH appear in the urine.

There is considerable evidence that GH exerts metabolic effects in humans that continue after cessation of linear growth, including effects on body composition [76], serum lipids, insulin status (insulin-like and insulin-antagonistic effects) [77,78], bone turnover (increases bone mass, mineral content, and the number of bone modeling units) [79,80], and physical performance [81,82]. In addition, GH influences the homeostasis of water and electrolytes and interacts with the immune system [83]. In adipose tissue, GH leads to decreased glucose use and stimulation of lipolysis (hence insulin-antagonistic or diabetogenic effects) [84]. In the heart, skeletal muscle, and kidney, GH provokes glucose and amino acid uptake [85]. The anabolic actions of GH mostly are mediated through IGF-I and include increases in total body protein turnover and muscle synthesis. GH is at least as powerful as testosterone in this effect and, because they both operate through distinct pathways, their individual effects are additive and possibly synergistic. Hyposecretion of GH at an early age results in dwarfism, whereas GH hypersecretion occurring before or after puberty results in gigantism or acromegaly, respectively [86,87].

Adults who have GHD have been reported to have an increased risk for death from cardiovascular disease [88], reduced muscle mass and strength, lower bone density, and higher serum lipids than do adults who do not have GHD [81,82]. They also have been reported to have reduced energy, decreased vitality, poorer psychosocial adaptation, increased feelings of isolation, and other indices suggesting poor quality of life [81,82,89,90]. Although longitudinal studies of GH therapy for adults who have GHD showed improved clinical outcomes [91–93] and possibly lower mortality [94], there is little evidence of clinical benefit of GH therapy in the healthy elderly [20].

Growth hormone and exercise

Exercise is a potent stimulus for GH release [95–100]. The exercise-induced release of GH is influenced by many factors, including, but not limited to, the type, intensity, exercise duration, and training status of the participants. Because different investigators have used different experimental protocols and types of subjects, study result comparisons are difficult. Nevertheless, an increase in plasma GH stimulated by exercise has been well documented [95,96].

The exercise-induced release of GH is affected by gender. Women reach the maximal GH concentration faster than do men [101,102]; however, the relative increase in circulating GH is greater in men than in women, with the latter demonstrating higher maximal serum GH concentration because of greater resting levels in women [101,102].

In children, the release of GH in response to exercise increases with pubertal development in boys and girls. The administration of estrogen to prepubertal subjects increases the peak release of GH after exercise to pubertal levels, which strongly suggests that sex steroids stimulate the release of GH [103]. Coincidentally, the GH response to resistance exercise in women is greater during the luteal phase than during the follicular phase of the menstrual cycle [104].

The mechanisms responsible for the exercise-stimulated increase in GH remain unresolved. One hypothesis is that the activation of anaerobic glycolysis and the formation of lactate increase the release of GH [105]. It also is believed that the release of GH primarily is mediated through central cholinergic pathways [106] being augmented by pyridostigmine [107] and attenuated by atropine [108]. Peripheral metabolic signals also influence the GH response to exercise, with it being increased by fat intake and attenuated by carbohydrate ingestion [109–112].

Although it might be expected that the observed exercise-associated increase in GH would be paralleled by an increase in circulating IGF-I, study results to date conflict [113]. Some research groups have observed increments [114–119], others have observed no variations [120–125], and a decrease in IGF-I with exercise has been reported [126,127]. This may be due to differences in exercise type, intensity, duration and training status, individual nutritional and hormonal status variations, or technical differences in assay protocols.

Therapeutic use of growth hormone

The US Food and Drug Administration (FDA) has approved the use of GH in children for the treatment of growth failure secondary to GHD, chronic renal failure, Turner syndrome, Prader-Willi syndrome, persistent growth failure following intrauterine growth retardation, and idiopathic short stature. In adults, FDA-approved use is indicated in GHD and AIDS wasting syndrome. Nonconventional uses of GH therapy in children include achondroplasia and hypochondroplasia, dysmorphic syndromes, cystic fibrosis, juvenile chronic arthritis, short bowel disease, congenital adrenal hyperplasia, and burns [128].

The use of GH in adults who have GHD is based on evidence that GH can reverse some of the abnormalities common in this population. These abnormalities include changes in body composition (increased total body fat, decreased lean body mass) [129–132], worsening of lipoprotein profile, and impaired ventilatory function [81,82,130–134]. In addition, studies have demonstrated an increase in hemoglobin concentration [135,136] and improvements in wound healing and ligamentous strength [132], bone mineral density, strength [137–141], cardiac function [142,143], and quality of life in adult patients who have GHD and are treated with GH [144].

Dosing and cost

In children who have GHD, GH is prescribed in doses that are considered physiologic, so that they may achieve a height within the range of their genetic potential [144]. The mean duration of therapy for this indication is 4 to 7 years [145]. Although long-term data about GH therapy for adults is not available, it is suggested to be life-long [146].

Dosing plans have evolved from weight-based to individualized dose-titration strategies, with final maintenance doses being lower in the latter scenario [147,148].

Although suggested dosages vary, all sources recommend a low starting dose with a gradual increase to a maintenance dose [144]. The maintenance dose typically is higher in women than in men [149,150] and is higher still in women receiving oral estrogen replacement [151]. GH secretion normally decreases with age, and older patients have an increased susceptibility to GH-related side effects [41]. Therefore, GH dosing should be lower in older patients. By the same token, higher doses may be appropriate in some transition and young adult patients [152]. Available from several pharmaceutical companies, current preparations of rhGH have a biopotency of 3 IU/mg, using the World Health Organization reference preparation 88/624. In prepubertal children, GH is used routinely in the range of 25 to 50 μg/kg/d [153,154]. Doses as high as 100 μg/kg/d have been used in pubertal children who have GHD [155]. In adults, it is recommended that therapy start with a low dose of around 0.15 to 0.30 mg/d (0.45–0.90 IU/d). Additionally, although the maintenance dose may vary considerably from person to person, it seldom exceeds 1.0 mg/d (3 IU/d) [156,157]. In accordance with the clinical practice of treating GH-deficient children, it is recommended that GH be administered through daily subcutaneous self-injections in the evening [48].

During GH treatment, patients should be monitored at 1- to 2-month intervals during dose titration and semiannually thereafter. Such monitoring should include a clinical evaluation, an assessment of side effects, and measurement of IGF-I levels. The lipid profile and a fasting glucose should be assessed annually. Assessment of quality of life also is used for monitoring the response to therapy [152,158]. In children, the response to therapy is monitored by following growth curves carefully and by monitoring radiographic bone age. Peak bone mass generally has not been achieved at the time that final height is attained. Therefore, monitoring bone mineral density before discontinuation of GH therapy should be considered.

GH is expensive, and the estimated annual cost depends on dose, frequency, and the proprietary preparation used [159,160]. The annual estimated cost of GH treatment for a 30-kg child is approximately $20,000 [161].

Growth hormone as a doping agent

Despite the lack of evidence supporting significant positive effects of GH as an ergogenic aid, there are underground reports of the abuse of GH by athletes and bodybuilders for its anabolic properties. Such abuse rests on the belief that GH augments performance in endurance and power sports, is hard to detect [36], and is without major side effects [162,163]. In addition, it is believed that GH strengthens tendons and ligaments, prevents stress fractures, and speeds the healing process [23]. Among bodybuilders striving to achieve the "ripped look," GH misuse is believed to decrease the subcutaneous fat through a repartitioning effect and to promote hypertrophy of their muscle fibers [162,164]. Although it is unknown how popular GH is among female athletes, its appeal stems from the lower risk for androgenic side effects than are seen with anabolic steroids. Moreover, its use for endurance sports, in combination with erythropoietin as a method for enhancing oxygen transport, is gaining popularity; however, the few controlled studies involving supraphysiologic doses of GH to athletes have failed to show significant positive effects [162,165–171].

The applicability of these studies to a potential ergogenic effect in elite competitive sports may be limited. Athletes are highly trained to know their performance and to evaluate small changes in response to changes in training. At elite competitive levels, the differences in performance required to win can be measured in fractions of a percent, whereas clinical trials are designed to evaluate large changes because of their small sample sizes [162]. The durations of the studies were short to assess any improvements, especially given that athletes likely would take GH for prolonged periods in cycles lasting for 6 to 12 weeks or longer [59]. Moreover, the doses of GH used in studies, although supraphysiologic, were low. Underground reports mention that athletes take much larger doses of up to 25 IU/d [36], with a cost from $3000 to $5000 per month [172]. In addition, no study has evaluated the use of a combination of GH and anabolic steroids in power sports or GH and erythropoietin in endurance sports, which are theorized to be synergistic in their action [173].

Adverse effects of growth hormone

The short- and long-term risks of GH use in athletic training are not well known because epidemiologic data are lacking. There is evidence that acute administration of rhGH results in exaggerated increases in plasma lactate and glycerol as well as serum fatty acids in endurance-trained athletes. The increase in plasma lactate has been hypothesized to explain the decrease in exercise performance observed in these athletes [174]; however, a bigger danger probably is the exaggerated high fatty acidemia resulting from the additive effects of the acute rhGH administration and exercise on lipolysis, which could promote cardiac arrhythmias [164]. Moreover, the chronic abuse of supraphysiologic doses of GH in athletics is likely to be associated with significant side effects, as illustrated by studies of acromegalic patients [175–180]. Table 1 describes the potential side effects associated with GH supplementation in athletes. The adverse effects of GH therapy occur in fewer than 3% of treated children compared to approximately 10% of adults using therapeutic doses that are much lower than what athletes might use without supervision.

Detection of growth hormone doping

Until the 2004 Olympic Games in Athens, rhGH doping was considered undetectable. The difficulty of providing court evidence of the illegal use of GH derives mainly from its biochemical properties. The amino acid sequence

Table 1
Potential side effects of growth hormone misuse in athletes

Cardiovascular	Hypertension, cardiomyopathy, congestive heart failure, arrhythmia
Pulmonary	Respiratory failure, sleep apnea, narcolepsy, sleep disturbances
Musculoskeletal	Osteoarthritis, carpal tunnel syndrome, slipped capital femoral epiphysis, worsening of existing scoliosis, osteoporosis, arthralgias, muscle weakness, myopathy, avascular necrosis of the femoral head, gigantism
Endocrine and metabolic	Diabetes mellitus, insulin resistance, glucose intolerance, dyslipidemia, peripheral edema, hypothyroidism, menstrual irregularity, erectile dysfunction, multiple endocrine neoplasia type 1 (for those who have a genetic mutation)
Neurologic	Idiopathic intracranial hypertension (pseudotumor cerebri), visual field defects, cranial nerve palsy, headache
Malignancy	Increased risk of leukemia, solid tumors (breast, colon, prostate, and endometrial cancer), and increased risk of second neoplasms
Infection	HIV/AIDS, hepatitis B and C (nonsterile or contaminated syringes), Creutzfeldt-Jakob disease (GH extracted from human pituitary glands obtained on the "black market")
Cosmetic	Prognathism and jaw malocclusion, coarsened facial appearance, increased skull circumference, dentition problems, acral overgrowth, frontal bone bossing, gynecomastia
Visceromegaly	Tongue, thyroid gland, salivary glands, liver, spleen, kidney, prostate
Skin and gastrointestinal	Hyperhydrosis, oily texture, skin tags, colon polyps
Injection injuries	Direct and indirect trauma to nerves and soft tissue, abscess
Other	Counterfeit products (unable to advise on the relative safety of each product), compromised quality of life, increased mortality

Data from Refs. [116,164,174–192].

of the recombinant molecule is identical to the major 22-kd isoform secreted by the pituitary gland. In addition, the high intraindividual and interindividual variability in secretion makes it difficult to detect doping.

To overcome these problems, two independent approaches have been devised based on the use of blood samples to develop a valid test. The first has been the development of double immunologic tests: one preferentially recognizes 22-kd GH, and the other recognizes all other isoforms secreted by the pituitary gland [193]. Thus, the administration of GH increases the relative abundance of the 22-kd GH major isoform over all other circulating forms. When the ratio between the two proportions is calculated, it differs from that seen when only pituitary-derived GH is present [36,193]. This test was used for the first time during the 2004 Olympics in Athens, with no samples declared positive [21]. The lack of positive findings may result from this test's short window of detection, believed to be approximately 24 hours after injection. After this time, no rhGH will be detected in the circulation, and levels of the two GH forms will return to normal [194]. Hence, this method is best suited for "out of competition" testing, when an unannounced blood sample might be taken within 24 hours of the last rhGH injection [59].

The second approach relies on the analysis of more stable serum variables implied in the biologic cascade produced by GH secretion or doping application. These include combining measurements of IGF-I, IGFBP-3, and the acid-labile subunit as markers of acute GH "doping" [195] and using markers of collagen and bone turnover [196], such as N-terminal peptide of type III procollagen, collagen I C-terminal telopeptide, osteocalcin, and collagen I C-terminal propeptide [197,198]. These markers are similar to those that have been reported to be elevated in acromegaly [199,200]. These tests have the advantage of using stable variables with a much longer half-life than hGH, so that the "window of opportunity" (days or months) varies in relation to the extent and duration of abuse. Thus, this antidoping approach would be best suited for postcompetition samples [85]. Although promising, this approach requires the construction of a reference range of markers in plasma of elite athletes from different ethnicities and sport disciplines [201], a dataset that is unavailable [162].

Urine samples are used most frequently for doping analyses. Because GH has a short half-life in the circulation [202], the analysis of urine samples could provide a longer opportunity of time for a "diagnostic window." The problem is that the average urine concentration of GH is between 100 and 1000 times less than in blood, and the complex molecular changes resulting from the renal excretion process are not understood well enough to provide a meaningful evaluation [203,204].

Although attention currently is focused on the ergogenic properties of GH, there is evidence that other components of the hypothalamic-pituitary-IGF-I axis also are being abused. IGF-I, in particular, is associated with several specific side effects, in addition to those common to GH. These include severe lipodystrophy (if injected repeatedly at the same site); enlargement of the spleen, kidney, and lymphoid tissue; and severe hypoglycemia [204].

Another potential way GH circulatory levels are increased while circumventing standard detection methods is by using GH secretagogues (GHSs). GHSs are synthetic molecules that stimulate and amplify pulsatile pituitary GH release by way of a separate pathway distinct from GHRH/SRIH. Various GHSs can be used intravenously, subcutaneously, intranasally, or orally. Examples of GHSs include GHRP-1, hexarelin, MK-0677, SM-130686, and EP-01572 [205].

Studies suggest that youth are not likely to volunteer information about drug or supplement use to health professionals [206]. Consequently, it is important to screen routinely for performance-enhancing substances during office visits and preparticipation physicals. When young people do admit use of these substances, they should be queried regarding the reasons, dosing, and frequency of use. Additionally, information regarding the substance's source and cost should be obtained. This is important because illegally obtained substances have the additional risk of being counterfeit products with unsafe components. Some athletes may be purchasing the cheaper, black market GH extracted from human pituitary glands. Produced in this way, GH is associated with the potential transmission of diseases. To gain the confidence of the young person, the health provider should be able to openly discuss the perceived performance effects as well as the adverse effects, including what is and is not known about a given substance. The provider should explain that lack of information does not imply safety. It should also be acknowledged that benefits occur for those who are deficient in GH, but are much less certain for normal individuals, even at high doses, which increase the risk of side effects. Healthy ways to improve sports performance and appearance should be discussed with youth.

Approaches to combat the use of drugs by young athletes generally have involved changes in rules and testing and preventative educational initiatives [207]. Some schools use drug testing of high school athletes [208]; however, the GH testing is complex and is unlikely to be implemented in high schools in the near future. A more promising approach to combating youth drug use in sports may be educational programs that are designed to teach students about the facts and the myths of these substances. Examples of such interventions include the Adolescent Training and Learning to Avoid Steroids Program for boys [209,210] and Athletes Targeting Healthy Exercise and Nutrition Alternatives Program for girls [211]. It is important that educational programs include information on the dangers of these drugs from a medical perspective as well as the value of making good decisions and playing by the rules.

Summary

The underground abuse of GH among young athletes presents a challenge to medical professionals. Health care professionals providing knowledgeable guidance regarding healthy ways to improve performance and appearance, as well as accurate information regarding the substances' perceived benefits, risks, and unknown qualities, is invaluable to the young athlete. Further research focused on the profile and motivation of young people who use GH is essential to understanding and better intervening with those who use these substances.

Acknowledgments

The author gratefully acknowledges critical assistance from Teresa N. D. Buzzini, PsyD, and pediatric endocrinologist John J. Jaramillo, MD.

References

[1] Chinese swimmer's bag held banned hormone. New York Times. January 10, 1998. p. C-2.

[2] Aussies fine Stallone over growth hormone. The Albuquerque Tribune. May 22, 2007. p. A-6.

[3] Campbell D. Growth drug that put out Olympic flame. The Observer. September 10, 2000; section 18–19.

[4] Curry J. Pitcher used human growth hormone. New York Times. June 7, 2006. p. D-3.

[5] Fainaru-Wada M, Williams L. Sprinter admitted to use of BALCO 'magic potion.' San Francisco Chronicle. June 24, 2004.

[6] Fainaru-Wada M, Williams L. Giambi admitted taking steroids. San Francisco Chronicle. December 2, 2004; section A-1.

[7] Hall C. Doping for gold. San Francisco Chronicle. September 11, 2000; section A-6.

[8] Lemonick M. Le tour des drugs. Time. August 10, 1998. p. 76.

[9] Mackay D. How HGH cheats hit the end of the line. The Guardian. July 28, 2004.

[10] Reynolds G. Raging hormones. New York Times. August 20, 2006.

[11] Samuel A. Tour de France steadfast in ouster of Festina team. New York Times. July 19, 1998. p. A-1.

[12] Evans H, Long J. The effect of the anterior lobe administered intraperitoneally upon growth, maturity, and oestrus cycles of the rat [abstract]. Anat Rec 1921;21:62.

[13] Engelbach W, Schaeffer R, Brosius W. Endocrine growth deficiencies: diagnosis and treatment. Endocrinology 1933;17:250.

[14] Li C, Evans H. Isolation of pituitary growth hormone. Science 1944;99:183–4.

[15] Li CH, Papkoff H. Preparation and properties of growth hormone from human and monkey pituitary glands. Science 1956;124(3235):1293–4.

[16] Raben MS. Treatment of a pituitary dwarf with human growth hormone. J Clin Endocrinol Metab 1958;18(8):901–3.

[17] Underwood LE, Fisher DA, Frasier SD, et al. Degenerative neurologic disease in patients formerly treated with human growth hormone: Report of the Committee on Growth Hormone Use of the Lawson Wilkins Pediatric Endocrine Society, May 1985. J Pediatr 1985; 107(1):10–2.

[18] Grumbach MM, Bin-Abbas BS, Kaplan SL. The growth hormone cascade: progress and long-term results of growth hormone treatment in growth hormone deficiency. Horm Res 1998;49(Suppl 2):41–57.

[19] Fradkin JE, Schonberger LB, Mills JL, et al. Creutzfeldt-Jakob disease in pituitary growth hormone recipients in the United States. JAMA 1991;265(7):880–4.

[20] Liu H, Bravata DM, Olkin I, et al. Systematic review: the safety and efficacy of growth hormone in the healthy elderly. Ann Intern Med 2007;146(2):104–15.

[21] Saugy M, Robinson N, Saudan C, et al. Human growth hormone doping in sport. Br J Sports Med 2006;40(Suppl 1) i35–9.

[22] Kicman AT, Cowan DA. Peptide hormones and sport: misuse and detection. Br Med Bull 1992;48(3):496–517.

[23] Duchaine D. Underground steroid handbook. 1st edition. Venice (CA): HLR Technical Books; 1983.

[24] NCAA. NCAA study of substance use habits of college student athletes; 2001. Available at: http://www.ncaa.org/library/research/substance_use_habits/2001/substance_use_habits.pdf. Accessed June 13, 2007.

[25] Rickert VI, Pawlak-Morello C, Sheppard V, et al. Human growth hormone: a new substance of abuse among adolescents? Clin Pediatr 1992;31(12):723–6.

[26] Hirt H, Kimelman J, Birnbaum MJ, et al. The human growth hormone gene locus: structure, evolution, and allelic variations. DNA 1987;6(1):59–70.

[27] Healy ML, Russell-Jones D. Growth hormone and sport: abuse, potential benefits, and difficulties in detection. Br J Sports Med 1997;31(4):267–8.

[28] Frankenne F, Scippo ML, Van Beeumen J, et al. Identification of placental human growth hormone as the growth hormone-V gene expression product. J Clin Endocrinol Metab 1990;71(1):15–8.

[29] Eriksson L, Frankenne F, Eden S, et al. Growth hormone 24-h serum profiles during pregnancy–lack of pulsatility for the secretion of the placental variant. Br J Obstet Gynaecol 1989;96(8):949–53.

[30] de Zegher F, Vanderschueren-Lodeweyckx M, Spitz B, et al. Perinatal growth hormone (GH) physiology: effect of GH-releasing factor on maternal and fetal secretion of pituitary and placental GH. J Clin Endocrinol Metab 1990;71(2):520–2.

[31] Liu N, Mertani HC, Norstedt G, et al. Mode of the autocrine/paracrine mechanism of growth hormone action. Exp Cell Res 1997;237(1):196–206.

[32] Harvey S, Hull KL. Growth hormone. A paracrine growth factor? Endocrine 1997;7(3): 267–79.

[33] Boguszewski CL. Molecular heterogeneity of human GH: from basic research to clinical implications. J Endocrinol Invest 2003;26(3):274–88.

[34] Baumann G. Growth hormone heterogeneity in human pituitary and plasma. Horm Res 1999;51(Suppl 1):2–6.

[35] Lewis UJ, Sinha YN, Lewis GP. Structure and properties of members of the hGH family: a review. Endocr J 2000;47(Suppl):S1–8.

[36] Bidlingmaier M, Wu Z, Strasburger CJ. Test method: GH. Baillieres Best Pract Res 2000; 14(1):99–109.

[37] Baumann G. Growth hormone binding proteins and various forms of growth hormone: implications for measurements. Acta Paediatr Scand 1990;370:72–80 [discussion: 1].

[38] Muller EE, Locatelli V, Cocchi D. Neuroendocrine control of growth hormone secretion. Physiol Rev 1999;79(2):511–607.

[39] Kojima M, Hosoda H, Date Y, et al. Ghrelin is a growth-hormone-releasing acylated peptide from stomach. Nature 1999;402(6762):656–60.

[40] Tannenbaum GS, Epelbaum J, Bowers CY. Interrelationship between the novel peptide ghrelin and somatostatin/growth hormone-releasing hormone in regulation of pulsatile growth hormone secretion. Endocrinology 2003;144(3):967–74.

[41] Molitch ME, Clemmons DR, Malozowski S, et al. Evaluation and treatment of adult growth hormone deficiency: an Endocrine Society Clinical Practice Guideline. J Clin Endocrinol Metab 2006;91(5):1621–34.

[42] Ho KY, Evans WS, Blizzard RM, et al. Effects of sex and age on the 24-hour profile of growth hormone secretion in man: importance of endogenous estradiol concentrations. J Clin Endocrinol Metab 1987;64(1):51–8.

[43] Albertsson-Wikland K, Rosberg S, Karlberg J, et al. Analysis of 24-hour growth hormone profiles in healthy boys and girls of normal stature: relation to puberty. J Clin Endocrinol Metab 1994;78(5):1195–201.

[44] Stolar MW, Baumann G. Secretory patterns of growth hormone during basal periods in man. Metabolism 1986;35(9):883–8.

[45] Cappellin E, Gatti R, De Palo EF. Influence of gender in growth hormone status in adults: role of urinary growth hormone. Clin Chem 1999;45(3):443–4.

[46] Rogol AD, Martha P, Johnson M, et al. Growth hormone secretory dynamics during puberty. In: Adashi E, Thorner M, editors. The somatotrophic axis and the reproductive process in health and disease. New York: Springer-Verlag; 1995.

[47] Iranmanesh A, Lizarralde G, Veldhuis JD. Age and relative adiposity are specific negative determinants of the frequency and amplitude of growth hormone (GH) secretory bursts and the half-life of endogenous GH in healthy men. J Clin Endocrinol Metab 1991;73(5): 1081–8.

[48] Sonksen PH, Christiansen JS. Consensus guidelines for the diagnosis and treatment of adults with growth hormone deficiency. Growth Hormone Research Society. Growth Horm IGF Res 1998;8(Suppl B):89–92.

[49] Herington AC, Ymer S, Stevenson J. Identification and characterization of specific binding proteins for growth hormone in normal human sera. J Clin Invest 1986;77(6):1817–23.

[50] Baumann G, Stolar MW, Amburn K, et al. A specific growth hormone-binding protein in human plasma: initial characterization. J Clin Endocrinol Metab 1986;62(1):134–41.

[51] Leung DW, Spencer SA, Cachianes G, et al. Growth hormone receptor and serum binding protein: purification, cloning and expression. Nature 1987;330(6148):537–43.

[52] Leung KC, Doyle N, Ballesteros M, et al. Estrogen inhibits GH signaling by suppressing GH-induced JAK2 phosphorylation, an effect mediated by SOCS-2. Proc Natl Acad Sci U S A 2003;100(3):1016–21.

[53] Mullis PE, Wagner JK, Eble A, et al. Regulation of human growth hormone receptor gene transcription by human growth hormone binding protein. Mol Cell Endocrinol 1997; 131(1):89–96.

[54] Brown RJ, Adams JJ, Pelekanos RA, et al. Model for growth hormone receptor activation based on subunit rotation within a receptor dimer. Nat Struct Mol Biol 2005;12(9):814–21.

[55] Chen C, Brinkworth R, Waters MJ. The role of receptor dimerization domain residues in growth hormone signaling. J Biol Chem 1997;272(8):5133–40.

[56] Pearce KH Jr, Ultsch MH, Kelley RF, et al. Structural and mutational analysis of affinity-inert contact residues at the growth hormone-receptor interface. Biochemistry 1996;35(32): 10300–7.

[57] Goffin V, Shiverick KT, Kelly PA, et al. Sequence-function relationships within the expanding family of prolactin, growth hormone, placental lactogen, and related proteins in mammals. Endocr Rev 1996;17(4):385–410.

[58] Fuh G, Cunningham BC, Fukunaga R, et al. Rational design of potent antagonists to the human growth hormone receptor. Science 1992;256(5064):1677–80.

[59] Rigamonti AE, Cella SG, Marazzi N, et al. Growth hormone abuse: methods of detection. Trends Endocrinol Metab 2005;16(4):160–6.

[60] Martin JL, Coverley JA, Pattison ST, et al. Insulin-like growth factor-binding protein-3 production by MCF-7 breast cancer cells: stimulation by retinoic acid and cyclic adenosine monophosphate and differential effects of estradiol. Endocrinology 1995;136(3): 1219–26.

[61] Le Roith D. Seminars in medicine of the Beth Israel Deaconess Medical Center. Insulin-like growth factors. N Engl J Med 1997;336(9):633–40.

[62] O'Reilly KE, Rojo F, She QB, et al. mTOR inhibition induces upstream receptor tyrosine kinase signaling and activates Akt. Cancer Res 2006;66(3):1500–8.

[63] Fryburg DA, Jahn LA, Hill SA, et al. Insulin and insulin-like growth factor-I enhance human skeletal muscle protein anabolism during hyperaminoacidemia by different mechanisms. J Clin Invest 1995;96(4):1722–9.

[64] Butler AA, Le Roith D. Control of growth by the somatropic axis: growth hormone and the insulin-like growth factors have related and independent roles. Annu Rev Physiol 2001;63: 141–64.

[65] Le Roith D, Scavo L, Butler A. What is the role of circulating IGF-I? Trends Endocrinol Metab 2001;12(2):48–52.

[66] Clemmons DR. Quantitative measurement of IGF-I and its use in diagnosing and monitoring treatment of disorders of growth hormone secretion. Endocr Dev 2005;9:55–65.

[67] Butterfield GE, Thompson J, Rennie MJ, et al. Effect of rhGH and rhIGF-I treatment on protein utilization in elderly women. Am J Physiol 1997;272(1 Pt 1):E94–9.

[68] Brabant G, von zur Muhlen A, Wuster C, et al. Serum insulin-like growth factor I reference values for an automated chemiluminescence immunoassay system: results from a multicenter study. Horm Res 2003;60(2):53–60.

[69] Milani D, Carmichael JD, Welkowitz J, et al. Variability and reliability of single serum IGF-I measurements: impact on determining predictability of risk ratios in disease development. J Clin Endocrinol Metab 2004;89(5):2271–4.

[70] Parker ML, Utiger RD, Daughaday WH. Studies on human growth hormone. II. The physiological disposition and metabolic fate of human growth hormone in man. J Clin Invest 1962;41:262–8.

[71] Baumann G. Growth hormone binding protein 2001. J Pediatr Endocrinol Metab 2001; 14(4):355–75.

[72] Ho KY, Weissberger AJ, Stuart MC, et al. The pharmacokinetics, safety and endocrine effects of authentic biosynthetic human growth hormone in normal subjects. Clin Endocrinol (Oxf) 1989;30(4):335–45.

[73] van den Berg G, Veldhuis JD, Frolich M, et al. An amplitude-specific divergence in the pulsatile mode of growth hormone (GH) secretion underlies the gender difference in mean GH concentrations in men and premenopausal women. J Clin Endocrinol Metab 1996;81(7): 2460–7.

[74] Peacey SR, Toogood AA, Veldhuis JD, et al. The relationship between 24-hour growth hormone secretion and insulin-like growth factor I in patients with successfully treated acromegaly: impact of surgery or radiotherapy. J Clin Endocrinol Metab 2001;86(1): 259–66.

[75] Krogsgaard Thomsen M, Friis C, Sehested Hansen B, et al. Studies on the renal kinetics of growth hormone (GH) and on the GH receptor and related effects in animals. J Pediatr Endocrinol 1994;7(2):93–105.

[76] de Boer H, Blok GJ, Van der Veen EA. Clinical aspects of growth hormone deficiency in adults. Endocr Rev 1995;16(1):63–86.

[77] Tanner JW, Leingang KA, Mueckler MM, et al. Cellular mechanism of the insulin-like effect of growth hormone in adipocytes. Rapid translocation of the HepG2-type and adipocyte/muscle glucose transporters. Biochem J 1992;282(Pt 1):99–106.

[78] Fowelin J, Attvall S, von Schenck H, et al. Characterization of the insulin-antagonistic effect of growth hormone in man. Diabetologia 1991;34(7):500–6.

[79] Lissett CA, Shalet SM. Effects of growth hormone on bone and muscle. Growth Horm IGF Res 2000;10(Suppl B):S95–101.

[80] Nussey S, Whitehead S. Endocrinology: an integrated approach. London: BIOS Scientific Publishers Limited; 2001.

[81] Vance ML, Mauras N. Growth hormone therapy in adults and children. N Engl J Med 1999;341(16):1206–16.

[82] Carroll PV, Christ ER, Bengtsson BA, et al. Growth hormone deficiency in adulthood and the effects of growth hormone replacement: a review. Growth Hormone Research Society Scientific Committee. J Clin Endocrinol Metab 1998;83(2):382–95.

[83] Auernhammer CJ, Strasburger CJ. Effects of growth hormone and insulin-like growth factor I on the immune system. Eur J Endocrinol 1995;133(6):635–45.

[84] Samra JS, Clark ML, Humphreys SM, et al. Suppression of the nocturnal rise in growth hormone reduces subsequent lipolysis in subcutaneous adipose tissue. Eur J Clin Invest 1999;29(12):1045–52.

[85] Sonksen PH. Insulin, growth hormone and sport. J Endocrinol 2001;170(1):13–25.

[86] Ohlsson C, Bengtsson BA, Isaksson OG, et al. Growth hormone and bone. Endocr Rev 1998;19(1):55–79.

[87] Melmed S. Acromegaly. N Engl J Med 1990;322(14):966–77.

[88] American Academy of Pediatrics Committee on Drugs and Committee on Bioethics. Considerations related to the use of recombinant human growth hormone in children. Pediatrics 1997;99(1):122–9.

[89] Badia X, Lucas A, Sanmarti A, et al. One-year follow-up of quality of life in adults with untreated growth hormone deficiency. Clin Endocrinol (Oxf) 1998;49(6):765–71.

[90] Dean HJ, McTaggart TL, Fish DG, et al. The educational, vocational, and marital status of growth hormone-deficient adults treated with growth hormone during childhood. Am J Dis Child 1985;139(11):1105–10.

[91] Baum HB, Biller BM, Finkelstein JS, et al. Effects of physiologic growth hormone therapy on bone density and body composition in patients with adult-onset growth hormone deficiency. A randomized, placebo-controlled trial. Ann Intern Med 1996;125(11): 883–90.

[92] Biller BM, Sesmilo G, Baum HB, et al. Withdrawal of long-term physiological growth hormone (GH) administration: differential effects on bone density and body composition in men with adult-onset GH deficiency. J Clin Endocrinol Metab 2000;85(3):970–6.

[93] Feldt-Rasmussen U, Wilton P, Jonsson P. Aspects of growth hormone deficiency and replacement in elderly hypopituitary adults. Growth Horm IGF Res 2004;14(Suppl A):S51–8.

[94] Monson JP. Long-term experience with GH replacement therapy: efficacy and safety. Eur J Endocrinol 2003;148(Suppl 2):S9–14.

[95] Flanagan DE, Taylor MC, Parfitt V, et al. Urinary growth hormone following exercise to assess growth hormone production in adults. Clin Endocrinol (Oxf) 1997;46(4):425–9.

[96] Galbo H. The hormonal response to exercise. Proc Nutr Soc 1985;44(2):257–66.

[97] Kraemer RR, Blair MS, McCaferty R, et al. Running-induced alterations in growth hormone, prolactin, triiodothyronine, and thyroxine concentrations in trained and untrained men and women. Res Q Exerc Sport 1993;64(1):69–74.

[98] Snegovskaya V, Viru A. Steroid and pituitary hormone responses to rowing: relative significance of exercise intensity and duration and performance level. Eur J Appl Physiol Occup Physiol 1993;67(1):59–65.

[99] Snegovskaya V, Viru A. Elevation of cortisol and growth hormone levels in the course of further improvement of performance capacity in trained rowers. Int J Sports Med 1993; 14(4):202–6.

[100] Weltman JY, Weltman AF, van der Heijden M, et al. Effect of intensity of exercise on 24-hour growth hormone (GH) release. Med Sci Sports Exerc 1994;26(Suppl 5):S37.

[101] Bunt JC, Boileau RA, Bahr JM, et al. Sex and training differences in human growth hormone levels during prolonged exercise. J Appl Physiol 1986;61(5):1796–801.

[102] Wideman L, Weltman JY, Shah N, et al. Effects of gender on exercise-induced growth hormone release. J Appl Physiol 1999;87(3):1154–62.

[103] Marin G, Domene HM, Barnes KM, et al. The effects of estrogen priming and puberty on the growth hormone response to standardized treadmill exercise and arginine-insulin in normal girls and boys. J Clin Endocrinol Metab 1994;79(2):537–41.

[104] Kraemer RR, Heleniak RJ, Tryniecki JL, et al. Follicular and luteal phase hormonal responses to low-volume resistive exercise. Med Sci Sports Exerc 1995;27(6):809–17.

[105] Gordon SE, Kraemer WJ, Vos NH, et al. Effect of acid-base balance on the growth hormone response to acute high-intensity cycle exercise. J Appl Physiol 1994;76(2):821–9.

[106] Thompson DL, Weltman JY, Rogol AD, et al. Cholinergic and opioid involvement in release of growth hormone during exercise and recovery. J Appl Physiol 1993;75(2):870–8.

[107] Cappa M, Grossi A, Benedetti S, et al. Effect of the enhancement of the cholinergic tone by pyridostigmine on the exercise-induced growth hormone release in man. J Endocrinol Invest 1993;16(6):421–4.

[108] Brillon D, Nabil N, Jacobs LS. Cholinergic but not serotonergic mediation of exercise-induced growth hormone secretion. Endocr Res 1986;12(2):137–46.

[109] Galbo H, Holst JJ, Christensen NJ. The effect of different diets and of insulin on the hormonal response to prolonged exercise. Acta Physiol Scand 1979;107(1):19–32.

[110] Johannessen A, Hagen C, Galbo H. Prolactin, growth hormone, thyrotropin, 3,5,3'-triiodothyronine, and thyroxine responses to exercise after fat- and carbohydrate-enriched diet. J Clin Endocrinol Metab 1981;52(1):56–61.

[111] Nieman DC, Nehlsen-Cannarella SL, Fagoaga OR, et al. Influence of mode and carbohydrate on the cytokine response to heavy exertion. Med Sci Sports Exerc 1998;30(5): 671–8.

[112] Tsintzas OK, Williams C, Wilson W, et al. Influence of carbohydrate supplementation early in exercise on endurance running capacity. Med Sci Sports Exerc 1996;28(11):1373–9.

[113] Jenkins PJ. Growth hormone and exercise. Clin Endocrinol (Oxf) 1999;50(6):683–9.

[114] Bang P, Brandt J, Degerblad M, et al. Exercise-induced changes in insulin-like growth factors and their low molecular weight binding protein in healthy subjects and patients with growth hormone deficiency. Eur J Clin Invest 1990;20(3):285–92.

[115] Cappon J, Brasel JA, Mohan S, et al. Effect of brief exercise on circulating insulin-like growth factor I. J Appl Physiol 1994;76(6):2490–6.

[116] Deyssig R, Frisch H. Self-administration of cadaveric growth hormone in power athletes. Lancet 1993;341(8847):768–9.

[117] Kraemer WJ, Fleck SJ, Dziados JE, et al. Changes in hormonal concentrations after different heavy-resistance exercise protocols in women. J Appl Physiol 1993;75(2):594–604.

[118] Kraemer WJ, Marchitelli L, Gordon SE, et al. Hormonal and growth factor responses to heavy resistance exercise protocols. J Appl Physiol 1990;69(4):1442–50.

[119] Schwarz AJ, Brasel JA, Hintz RL, et al. Acute effect of brief low- and high-intensity exercise on circulating insulin-like growth factor (IGF) I, II, and IGF-binding protein-3 and its proteolysis in young healthy men. J Clin Endocrinol Metab 1996;81(10):3492–7.

[120] Di Luigi L, Conti FG, Casini A, et al. Growth hormone and insulin-like growth factor I responses to moderate submaximal acute physical exercise in man: effects of octreotide, a somatostatin analogue, administration. Int J Sports Med 1997;18(4):257–63.

[121] Hellenius ML, Brismar KE, Berglund BH, et al. Effects on glucose tolerance, insulin secretion, insulin-like growth factor 1 and its binding protein, IGFBP-1, in a randomized controlled diet and exercise study in healthy, middle-aged men. J Intern Med 1995;238(2): 121–30.

[122] Hopkins NJ, Jakeman PM, Hughes SC, et al. Changes in circulating insulin-like growth factor-binding protein-1 (IGFBP-1) during prolonged exercise: effect of carbohydrate feeding. J Clin Endocrinol Metab 1994;79(6):1887–90.

[123] Jahreis G, Hesse V, Schmidt HE, et al. Effect of endurance exercise on somatomedin-C/insulin-like growth factor I concentration in male and female runners. Exp Clin Endocrinol 1989;94(1–2):89–96.

[124] Kraemer WJ, Aguilera BA, Terada M, et al. Responses of IGF-I to endogenous increases in growth hormone after heavy-resistance exercise. J Appl Physiol 1995;79(4):1310–5.

[125] Sartorio A, Marazzi N, Agosti F, et al. Elite volunteer athletes of different sport disciplines may have elevated baseline GH levels divorced from unaltered levels of both IGF-I and GH-dependent bone and collagen markers: a study on-the-field. J Endocrinol Invest 2004;27(5):410–5.

[126] Eliakim A, Brasel JA, Barstow TJ, et al. Peak oxygen uptake, muscle volume, and the growth hormone-insulin-like growth factor-I axis in adolescent males. Med Sci Sports Exerc 1998;30(4):512–7.

[127] Eliakim A, Brasel JA, Mohan S, et al. Physical fitness, endurance training, and the growth hormone-insulin-like growth factor I system in adolescent females. J Clin Endocrinol Metab 1996;81(11):3986–92.

[128] Cappa M, Ubertini G, Colabianchi D, et-al. Non-conventional use of growth hormone therapy. Acta Paediatr Suppl;95(452):9–13.

[129] Gibney J, Wallace JD, Spinks T, et al. The effects of 10 years of recombinant human growth hormone (GH) in adult GH-deficient patients. J Clin Endocrinol Metab 1999;84(8): 2596–602.

[130] Jorgensen JO, Thuesen L, Muller J, et al. Three years of growth hormone treatment in growth hormone-deficient adults: near normalization of body composition and physical performance. Eur J Endocrinol 1994;130(3):224–8.

[131] Jorgensen JO, Vahl N, Hansen TB, et al. Growth hormone versus placebo treatment for one year in growth hormone deficient adults: increase in exercise capacity and normalization of body composition. Clin Endocrinol (Oxf) 1996;45(6):681–8.

[132] Salomon F, Cuneo RC, Hesp R, et al. The effects of treatment with recombinant human growth hormone on body composition and metabolism in adults with growth hormone deficiency. N Engl J Med 1989;321(26):1797–803.

[133] Barkan AL, Clemmons DR, Molitch ME, et al. Growth hormone therapy for hypopituitary adults: time for re-appraisal. Trends Endocrinol Metab 2000;11(6):238–45.

[134] Merola B, Longobardi S, Sofia M, et al. Lung volumes and respiratory muscle strength in adult patients with childhood- or adult-onset growth hormone deficiency: effect of 12 months' growth hormone replacement therapy. Eur J Endocrinol 1996;135(5):553–8.

[135] Christ ER, Cummings MH, Westwood NB, et al. The importance of growth hormone in the regulation of erythropoiesis, red cell mass, and plasma volume in adults with growth hormone deficiency. J Clin Endocrinol Metab 1997;82(9):2985–90.

[136] Ten Have SM, van der Lely AJ, Lamberts SW. Increase in haemoglobin concentrations in growth hormone deficient adults during human recombinant growth hormone replacement therapy. Clin Endocrinol (Oxf) 1997;47(5):565–70.

[137] Cuneo RC, Salomon F, Wiles CM, et al. Growth hormone treatment in growth hormone-deficient adults. II. Effects on exercise performance. J Appl Physiol 1991;70(2):695–700.

[138] Cuneo RC, Salomon F, Wiles CM, et al. Growth hormone treatment in growth hormone-deficient adults. I. Effects on muscle mass and strength. J Appl Physiol 1991;70(2):688–94.

[139] Beshyah SA, Freemantle C, Shahi M, et al. Replacement treatment with biosynthetic human growth hormone in growth hormone-deficient hypopituitary adults. Clin Endocrinol (Oxf) 1995;42(1):73–84.

[140] Jorgensen JO, Pedersen SA, Thuesen L, et al. Long-term growth hormone treatment in growth hormone deficient adults. Acta Endocrinol (Copenh) 1991;125(5):449–53.

[141] Rodriguez-Arnao J, Jabbar A, Fulcher K, et al. Effects of growth hormone replacement on physical performance and body composition in GH deficient adults. Clin Endocrinol (Oxf) 1999;51(1):53–60.

[142] Cittadini A, Cuocolo A, Merola B, et al. Impaired cardiac performance in GH-deficient adults and its improvement after GH replacement. Am J Physiol 1994;267(2 Pt 1):E219–25.

[143] Cuneo RC, Salomon F, Wilmshurst P, et al. Cardiovascular effects of growth hormone treatment in growth-hormone-deficient adults: stimulation of the renin-aldosterone system. Clin Sci (Lond) 1991;81(5):587–92.

[144] Radcliffe DJ, Pliskin JS, Silvers JB, et al. Growth hormone therapy and quality of life in adults and children. Pharmacoeconomics 2004;22(8):499–524.

[145] Bryant J, Cave C, Mihaylova B, et al. Clinical effectiveness and cost-effectiveness of growth hormone in children: a systematic review and economic evaluation. Health Technol Assess 2002;6(18):1–168.

[146] Gharib H, Cook DM, Saenger PH, et al. American Association of Clinical Endocrinologists medical guidelines for clinical practice for growth hormone use in adults and children–2003 update. Endocr Pract 2003;9(1):64–76.

[147] Hoffman AR, Strasburger CJ, Zagar A, et al. Efficacy and tolerability of an individualized dosing regimen for adult growth hormone replacement therapy in comparison with fixed body weight-based dosing. J Clin Endocrinol Metab 2004;89(7):3224–33.

[148] Johannsson G, Rosen T, Bengtsson BA. Individualized dose titration of growth hormone (GH) during GH replacement in hypopituitary adults. Clin Endocrinol (Oxf) 1997;47(5):571–81.

[149] Burman P, Johansson AG, Siegbahn A, et al. Growth hormone (GH)-deficient men are more responsive to GH replacement therapy than women. J Clin Endocrinol Metab 1997;82(2):550–5.

[150] Drake WM, Coyte D, Camacho-Hubner C, et al. Optimizing growth hormone replacement therapy by dose titration in hypopituitary adults. J Clin Endocrinol Metab 1998;83(11): 3913–9.

[151] Cook DM, Ludlam WH, Cook MB. Route of estrogen administration helps to determine growth hormone (GH) replacement dose in GH-deficient adults. J Clin Endocrinol Metab 1999;84(11):3956–60.

[152] Underwood LE, Attie KM, Baptista J. Growth hormone (GH) dose-response in young adults with childhood-onset GH deficiency: a two-year, multicenter, multiple-dose, placebo-controlled study. J Clin Endocrinol Metab 2003;88(11):5273–80.

[153] GH Research Society. Consensus guidelines for the diagnosis and treatment of growth hormone (GH) deficiency in childhood and adolescence: summary statement of the GH Research Society. J Clin Endocrinol Metab 2000;85(11):3990–3.

[154] Lee JM, Davis MM, Clark SJ, et al. Estimated cost-effectiveness of growth hormone therapy for idiopathic short stature. Arch Pediatr Adolesc Med 2006;160(3):263–9.

[155] Wilson TA, Rose SR, Cohen P, et al. Update of guidelines for the use of growth hormone in children: the Lawson Wilkins Pediatric Endocrinology Society Drug and Therapeutics Committee. J Pediatr 2003;143(4):415–21.

[156] Bengtsson BA, Eden S, Lonn L, et al. Treatment of adults with growth hormone (GH) deficiency with recombinant human GH. J Clin Endocrinol Metab 1993;76(2): 309–17.

[157] Rosen T, Johannsson G, Bengtsson BA. Consequences of growth hormone deficiency in adults, and effects of growth hormone replacement therapy. Acta Paediatr Suppl 1994; 399:21–4 [discussion: 5].

[158] Drake WM, Carroll PV, Maher KT, et al. The effect of cessation of growth hormone (GH) therapy on bone mineral accretion in GH-deficient adolescents at the completion of linear growth. J Clin Endocrinol Metab 2003;88(4):1658–63.

[159] Allen DB, Fost N. hGH for short stature: ethical issues raised by expanded access. J Pediatr 2004;144(5):648–52.

[160] Cuttler L, Silvers JB. Growth hormone treatment for idiopathic short stature: implications for practice and policy. Arch Pediatr Adolesc Med 2004;158(2):108–10.

[161] Growth hormone for normal short children. Med Lett Drugs Ther 2003;45(1169):89–90.

[162] Jenkins PJ. Growth hormone and exercise: physiology, use and abuse. Growth Horm IGF Res 2001;11(Suppl A):S71–7.

[163] van der Lely AJ. Hormone use and abuse: what is the difference between hormones as fountain of youth and doping in sports? J Endocrinol Invest 2003;26(9):932–6.

[164] Rennie MJ. Claims for the anabolic effects of growth hormone: a case of the emperor's new clothes? Br J Sports Med 2003;37(2):100–5.

[165] Crist DM, Peake GT, Egan PA, et al. Body composition response to exogenous GH during training in highly conditioned adults. J Appl Physiol 1988;65(2):579–84.

[166] Deyssig R, Frisch H, Blum WF, et al. Effect of growth hormone treatment on hormonal parameters, body composition and strength in athletes. Acta Endocrinol (Copenh) 1993; 128(4):313–8.

[167] Karila T, Koistinen H, Seppala M, et al. Growth hormone induced increase in serum IGFBP-3 level is reversed by anabolic steroids in substance abusing power athletes. Clin Endocrinol (Oxf) 1998;49(4):459–63.

[168] Pierard-Franchimont C, Henry F, Crielaard JM, et al. Mechanical properties of skin in recombinant human growth factor abusers among adult bodybuilders. Dermatology 1996; 192(4):389–92.

[169] Taaffe DR, Jin IH, Vu TH, et al. Lack of effect of recombinant human growth hormone (GH) on muscle morphology and GH-insulin-like growth factor expression in resistance-trained elderly men. J Clin Endocrinol Metab 1996;81(1):421–5.

[170] Yarasheski KE, Campbell JA, Smith K, et al. Effect of growth hormone and resistance exercise on muscle growth in young men. Am J Physiol 1992;262(3 Pt 1):E261–7.

[171] Yarasheski KE, Zachweija JJ, Angelopoulos TJ, et al. Short-term growth hormone treatment does not increase muscle protein synthesis in experienced weight lifters. J Appl Physiol 1993;74(6):3073–6.

[172] Koch JJ. Performance-enhancing: substances and their use among adolescent athletes. Pediatr Rev 2002;23(9):310–7.

[173] Schnirring L. Growth hormone doping: the search for a test. Phys Sportsmed 2000;28(4): 16–8.

[174] Lange KH, Larsson B, Flyvbjerg A, et al. Acute growth hormone administration causes exaggerated increases in plasma lactate and glycerol during moderate to high intensity bicycling in trained young men. J Clin Endocrinol Metab 2002;87(11):4966–75.

[175] Cittadini A, Berggren A, Longobardi S, et al. Supraphysiological doses of GH induce rapid changes in cardiac morphology and function. J Clin Endocrinol Metab 2002;87(4): 1654–9.

[176] Jenkins PJ, Fairclough PD, Richards T, et al. Acromegaly, colonic polyps and carcinoma. Clin Endocrinol (Oxf) 1997;47(1):17–22.

[177] Mastaglia FL, Barwich DD, Hall R. Myopathy in acromegaly. Lancet 1970;2(7679):907–9.

[178] Melmed S. Medical progress: acromegaly. N Engl J Med 2006;355(24):2558–73.

[179] Nabarro JD. Acromegaly. Clin Endocrinol (Oxf) 1987;26(4):481–512.

[180] Orme SM, McNally RJ, Cartwright RA, et al. Mortality and cancer incidence in acromegaly: a retrospective cohort study. United Kingdom Acromegaly Study Group. J Clin Endocrinol Metab 1998;83(8):2730–4.

[181] Allen NE, Roddam AW, Allen DS, et al. A prospective study of serum insulin-like growth factor-I (IGF-I), IGF-II, IGF-binding protein-3 and breast cancer risk. Br J Cancer 2005; 92(7):1283–7.

[182] Biermasz NR, Pereira AM, Smit JW, et al. Morbidity after long-term remission for acromegaly: persisting joint-related complaints cause reduced quality of life. J Clin Endocrinol Metab 2005;90(5):2731–9.

[183] Clayton PE, Cowell CT. Safety issues in children and adolescents during growth hormone therapy–a review. Growth Horm IGF Res 2000;10(6):306–17.

[184] Clayton RN. Cardiovascular function in acromegaly. Endocr Rev 2003;24(3):272–7.

[185] Colao A, Ferone D, Marzullo P, et al. Systemic complications of acromegaly: epidemiology, pathogenesis, and management. Endocr Rev 2004;25(1):102–52.

[186] Malozowski S, Stadel BV. Prepubertal gynecomastia during growth hormone therapy. J Pediatr 1995;126(4):659–61.

[187] Okasha M, Gunnell D, Holly J, et al. Childhood growth and adult cancer. Best Pract Res Clin Endocrinol Metab 2002;16(2):225–41.

[188] Perry JK, Emerald BS, Mertani HC, et al. The oncogenic potential of growth hormone. Growth Horm IGF Res 2006;16(5–6):277–89.

[189] Renehan AG, Shalet SM. Acromegaly and colorectal cancer: risk assessment should be based on population-based studies. J Clin Endocrinol Metab 2002;87(4):1909; author reply.

[190] Seminara S, Merello G, Masi S, et al. Effect of long-term growth hormone treatment on carbohydrate metabolism in children with growth hormone deficiency. Clin Endocrinol (Oxf) 1998;49(1):125–30.

[191] Swerdlow AJ, Higgins CD, Adlard P, et al. Risk of cancer in patients treated with human pituitary growth hormone in the UK, 1959–85: a cohort study. Lancet 2002;360(9329): 273–7.

[192] Takala J, Ruokonen E, Webster NR, et al. Increased mortality associated with growth hormone treatment in critically ill adults. N Engl J Med 1999;341(11):785–92.

[193] Wu Z, Bidlingmaier M, Dall R, et al. Detection of doping with human growth hormone. Lancet 1999;353(9156):895.

[194] Bidlingmaier M, Wu Z, Strasburger CJ. Problems with GH doping in sports. J Endocrinol Invest 2003;26(9):924–31.

[195] Wallace JD, Cuneo RC, Baxter R, et al. Detection of growth hormone abuse in athletes. Growth Horm IGF Res 1998;8(4):347–8.
[196] Wallace JD, Cuneo RC, Rosen T, et al. Bone markers and growth hormone (GH) abuse in athletes. Growth Horm IGF Res 1998;8(4):348.
[197] Longobardi S, Keay N, Ehrnborg C, et al. Growth hormone (GH) effects on bone and collagen turnover in healthy adults and its potential as a marker of GH abuse in sports: a double blind, placebo-controlled study. The GH-2000 Study Group. J Clin Endocrinol Metab 2000;85(4):1505–12.
[198] Wallace JD, Cuneo RC, Lundberg PA, et al. Responses of markers of bone and collagen turnover to exercise, growth hormone (GH) administration, and GH withdrawal in trained adult males. J Clin Endocrinol Metab 2000;85(1):124–33.
[199] Legovini P, De Menis E, Breda F, et al. Long-term effects of octreotide on markers of bone metabolism in acromegaly: evidence of increased serum parathormone concentrations. J Endocrinol Invest 1997;20(8):434–8.
[200] Piovesan A, Terzolo M, Reimondo G, et al. Biochemical markers of bone and collagen turnover in acromegaly or Cushing's syndrome. Horm Metab Res 1994;26(5):234–7.
[201] Ehrnborg C, Lange KH, Dall R, et al. The growth hormone/insulin-like growth factor-I axis hormones and bone markers in elite athletes in response to a maximum exercise test. J Clin Endocrinol Metab 2003;88(1):394–401.
[202] Holl RW, Schwarz U, Schauwecker P, et al. Diurnal variation in the elimination rate of human growth hormone (GH): the half-life of serum GH is prolonged in the evening, and affected by the source of the hormone, as well as by body size and serum estradiol. J Clin Endocrinol Metab 1993;77(1):216–20.
[203] Saugy M, Cardis C, Schweizer C, et al. Detection of human growth hormone doping in urine: out of competition tests are necessary. J Chromatogr 1996;687(1):201–11.
[204] Backeljauw PF, Underwood LE. Prolonged treatment with recombinant insulin-like growth factor-I in children with growth hormone insensitivity syndrome–a clinical research center study. GHIS Collaborative Group. J Clin Endocrinol Metab 1996;81(9):3312–7.
[205] Isidro ML, Cordido F. Growth hormone secretagogues. Comb Chem High Throughput Screen 2006;9(3):175–80.
[206] Kanayama G, Pope HG, Cohane G, et al. Risk factors for anabolic-androgenic steroid use among weightlifters: a case-control study. Drug Alcohol Depend 2003;71(1):77–86.
[207] Calfee R, Fadale P. Popular ergogenic drugs and supplements in young athletes. Pediatrics 2006;117(3):e577–89.
[208] National Federation of State High School Associations. Sports medicine: high school drug-testing programs: August 2003. Available at: www.nfhs.org. Accessed June 13, 2007.
[209] Goldberg L, Elliot D, Clarke GN, et al. Effects of a multidimensional anabolic steroid prevention intervention. The Adolescents Training and Learning to Avoid Steroids (ATLAS) Program. JAMA 1996;276(19):1555–62.
[210] Goldberg L, MacKinnon DP, Elliot DL, et al. The adolescents training and learning to avoid steroids program: preventing drug use and promoting health behaviors. Arch Pediatr Adolesc Med 2000;154(4):332–8.
[211] Elliot DL, Goldberg L, Moe EL, et al. Preventing substance use and disordered eating: initial outcomes of the ATHENA (athletes targeting healthy exercise and nutrition alternatives) program. Arch Pediatr Adolesc Med 2004;158(11):1043–9.

**ELSEVIER
SAUNDERS**

Pediatr Clin N Am 54 (2007) 845–851

PEDIATRIC CLINICS

OF NORTH AMERICA

Index

Note: Page numbers of article titles are in **boldface** type.

Moving?

Make sure your subscription moves with you!

To notify us of your new address, find your **Clinics Account Number** (located on your mailing label above your name), and contact customer service at:

E-mail: elspcs@elsevier.com

800-654-2452 (subscribers in the U.S. & Canada)
407-345-4000 (subscribers outside of the U.S. & Canada)

Fax number: 407-363-9661

Elsevier Periodicals Customer Service
6277 Sea Harbor Drive
Orlando, FL 32887-4800

*To ensure uninterrupted delivery of your subscription, please notify us at least 4 weeks in advance of move.